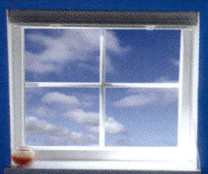

Heal your troubled mind

52 brilliant little ideas for tackling stress and defeating depression

Dr Sabina Dosani and Elisabeth Wilson

CAREFUL NOW

We hope that by reading the tips in this book you uncover some new ways to deal with your problems. However, we do not claim to have all the answers and we're certainly no substitute for doctors and mental health professionals. So if you are worried about your health, or that of somebody you love, please seek the advice of a professional first.

Copyright © The Infinite Ideas Company Ltd, 2007

The right of the contributors to be identified as the authors of this book has been asserted in accordance with the Copyright, Designs and Patents Act 1988.

First published in 2007 by
The Infinite Ideas Company Limited
36 St Giles
Oxford, OX1 3LD
United Kingdom
www.infideas.com

All rights reserved. Except for the quotation of small passages for the purposes of criticism or review, no part of this publication may be reproduced, stored in a retrieval system or transmitted in any form or by any means, electronic, mechanical, photocopying, recording, scanning or otherwise, except under the terms of the Copyright, Designs and Patents Act 1988 or under the terms of a licence issued by the Copyright Licensing Agency Ltd, 90 Tottenham Court Road, London W1T 4LP, UK, without the permission in writing of the publisher. Requests to the publisher should be addressed to the Permissions Department, Infinite Ideas Limited, 36 St Giles, Oxford, OX1 3LD, UK, or faxed to +44 (0)1865 514777.

A CIP catalogue record for this book is available from the British Library

ISBN 978-1-905940-04-2

Brand and product names are trademarks or registered trademarks of their respective owners.

Designed and typeset by Baseline Arts Ltd, Oxford
Printed in Singapore

Brilliant ideas

Introduction 11

1. Shrinks and quacks...................15
Lots of people claim they'll help you but check out their 'letters' to suss out what they can and can't do for you.

2. Run away... 17
. . . or to give it the grown-up name, retreat. Some time alone with your own thoughts is deeply relaxing.

3. Dear diary................................19
Try some free therapy. Writing a diary can be an oasis of serenity in your life and help you see what really matters.

4. Cherish yourself 21
We all know what we ought to do to relax but we often can't be bothered. Start taking relaxation seriously.

5. Listen up 23
The right music can move you from brow beaten to bouncy in just three minutes. Find your pearls of pop Prozac.

6. Aromatherapy?!.......................25
Yes, aromatherapy kicks ass, and it works. Try if for yourself – the proof of the pudding is in the eating.

7. Beat those blues 27
A little bit of what you fancy does you good so build some enjoyment into every day.

8. Perfect moments 29
If you develop the skill to create perfect moments, you'll guarantee that tomorrow will be less stressed than today.

9. It's your time 31
When you're feeling crushed by your things-to-do list, good time management can transform your mood and your life.

10. Don't act on impulse...............33
Focus, concentrate: stick to what you've started. That will cut your stress levels instantly.

11. **Counting sheep**..........35
Quality sleep is a serious depression buster. Here are some reliable routes to regular, refreshing rest.

12. **Out to get you**..........37
Are you ready for a journey to the weirder, wilder side? Relax. We're only talking a little white witchery.

13. **Drop if you stop?**..........39
If the lurgy blights the first week of your holiday, that's leisure sickness – 'stop and collapse' syndrome.

14. **Feeling SAD?**..........43
For many people, less daylight equals less happiness. Use these illuminating tips to avoid another winter of discontent.

15. **Your dark side**..........45
Reckon you're not an angry person? Maybe that's why you're so stressed.

16. **All in the mind**..........47
Ever wondered what's happening in your brain when you get depressed? This idea explains brain science.

17. **Learn to bounce**..........49
Everyone gets stressed but some people are better at dealing with it than others. That's because they're natural 'bouncers'.

18. **Go on, prove it**..........51
New miracle cures grace every health page, but which ones works? Here's a guide to help you sort fact from hype.

19. **Turning Japanese**..........53
Learn from Zen. The Japanese bath and tea ceremonies were as much about refreshing the spirit as cleansing the body.

20. **Magnetic attraction**..........55
Can magnets max your mood? Well, believe it or not, transcranial magnetic therapy has a lot going for it.

21. **Crisis management**..........57
Facing the week from hell? This is the toolbox for navigating through those really stressful, busy times.

22. **Get the cream**..........59
Wanna feel like the CAT that got the cream? You're just sixteen weeks from happiness with cognitive analytic therapy.

Brilliant ideas

23. **Restoration day**......................61
If you're suffering from chronic, long-term stress and burnout is imminent, here is your emergency plan.

24. **At the peak**............................63
High self-esteem makes you happier. Revving yours up should be easy if you follow these simple rules.

25. **The clinic is open**..................65
You know you're stressed and you know it's affecting your health. It's time to do something about it.

26. **Know what to do**....................67
Are you in need of ways to cope with problems that trigger depression? Try these tried and trusted strategies.

27. **How to be loved**.....................71
The need for approval can be a source of personal stress. Get a warm glow from dishing it out rather than seeking it.

28. **Don't panic**.............................73
Depression and anxiety go hand in glove. Fight back by managing panic attacks and all those irrational fears.

29. **Watch out: iceberg!**................75
Like the *Titanic*, you can be sailing true, then crunch! You're sunk. That's the effect of iceberg stress.

30. **Natural highs**.........................77
Poised to pop a herbal helper? The idea of nature's Prozac may be hard to swallow but it might just save your life.

31. **Stress is others** 79
Other people can sometimes leach the self-esteem out of you. Learn how to deal with these black holes.

32. **Just say no**.............................81
Are you a people pleaser, swamped by always saying 'yes'? Perfect the art of polite refusal and show depression the door.

33. **Conquer obstacles** 83
For every action, there's a payback. Work out the payback to drain away a lot of stress from a situation.

34. **Reboot**....................................85
What you think about what's happening affects the way you feel. A positive spin will improve your mood.

52 Brilliant Ideas – **Heal your troubled mind**

35. **Life-work balance**.................87
It should be life-work balance, not work-life. And that's what achieving it entails – a life-work.

36. **Rant and rave** 89
It's not getting angry that's the problem, it's how you express it. Gain advantage by transforming rage into passion.

37. **Speed parenting** 91
Children pick up adult stress like a dry sponge soaks up water. That's when you need focused parental skills.

38. **When drugs fail** 93
For a third of people, antidepressants don't work. If you're one of them, don't despair.

39. **Work to rules** 95
Take control. Don't let your working day be hijacked by others. The secret is to have your goals clearly in mind.

40. **Toil and trouble** 99
Work is often blamed for stressing us out. However, there's a flip side. Hard graft does have healing powers.

41. **Draw it out**.......................... 101
Lost for words? The answer could be to explore your thoughts and emotions using sketches, paints, clay etc.

42. **All hands on deck** 103
Having a regular massage can improve your quality of life and help you live with debilitating problems.

43. **Sexual healing** 105
Many depressed people lose interest in sex. Discover how to perk up your passions and your mood.

44. **Stress 'n' relax** 107
There's nothing wrong with stress: we're designed for it. The problem is how we deal with it.

45. **There for you** 109
Isolation worsens depression, but good friends can raise low moods. Discover the restorative powers of relationships.

46. **Time to play**.......................... 111
Picture what you'd do if you had a whole hour each day to yourself to spend doing exactly what you wanted.

Brilliant ideas

47. **Imagine**...................113
Visualisation means using your mind to create pictures. Use it to relax or prepare yourself for action.

48. **You're worth it**......................115
Down in the dumps with nothing to look forward too? Change that with some self-indulgent pampering.

49. **Shades of grey** 117
Depressed people think in all-or-nothing terms. Don't let self-imposed perfectionism make you feel you never measure up.

50. **Memory fix**...........................119
Never lose your keys again. Here's why stress eats your memory – and what you can do about it.

51. **A bright future**......................121
Sadly, once depression has paid you a visit, it's likely to return. Recognise its calling card and send it packing.

52. **On the shelf** 123
Find out what's in the pharm yard. Which drugs work; which make you feel worse; how can you tell the difference?

52 Brilliant Ideas – **Heal your troubled mind**

Brilliant ideas

Introduction

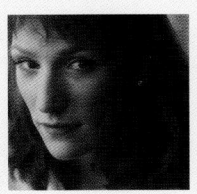

Stress and depression are linked. Stress can rewire your brain's emotional network leaving you stuck in repeated cycles of worry and misery. The hormones released by chronic stress can cause depression.

We all know that stress is a *bad thing*. It leaches our energy and is the forerunner of many of the major illnesses going. We also know that the ability to relax is a *good thing*, but, since you have to do it for yourself, the relaxation thing causes quite a few problems for us, too. It's yet another thing to add to the 'to-do' list, thereby adding to the pressure on your precious time – which adds to the stress. It can be all too easy to begin a descent into the depths of depression. That truly is not a good place to be.

This book is for people who are superbusy and for whom the usual advice doesn't ever hit. Let's face it, if you're the sort of time-rich person who already enjoys doing an hour of yoga every morning and then soaking for an hour in a candle-lit bath every night, you probably don't need any advice on destressing.

This book is for the people who struggle to find time for a shower, let alone a bath; the ones who are still clicking their mouse or ironing a shirt at 11.30 p.m; the ones (and there are many thousands of them) who don't take their full annual holiday leave and worry that stress is affecting their health and relationships (or they would do if they weren't so knackered and that report wasn't due in at 9 a.m.).

What we need are simple ways of dealing with stress that don't take much more effort than reading this book. And that's what you've got here. When you understand the impact of stress on your body, it's easier to take measures that disperse that stress. You'll become better at nipping the stressors in the bud – just as you nip the chances of getting dysentery in the bud by choosing not to drink dirty, smelly water.

Remember that stress *will* find you. Most of us can't avoid it. If we learn to relax, though, we can deal with it. If we don't learn in time, we can be tipped over the edge into full-on depression.

With depression, you need an even bigger first-aid kit to pull you through. In this book, we hope you'll find the basic tools to get you there, even when antidepressants don't work.

Brilliant ideas

When it comes to theory, we've been extremely promiscuous. Many of these ideas come from rival schools of therapy – tips from the mainstream sit alongside techniques from the fringes. No apologies. If any of the ideas work for you, add them to your depression-fighting arsenal.

If there is an apology to make, it'll be because – despite our best intentions – doctors' jargon has crept into the book. However, in the age of the Web and when so many people are taking antidepressants, it would have been crazy not to include something about how our brains work and how pharmaceuticals affect us. Depression is common (one in five women and one in ten men suffer from it) but everyone's depression is different. We don't know exactly how you feel, and we don't pretend to. We *do* know that defeating depression is often a long haul and we hope that this book helps you take the ride in your stride.

52 Brilliant Ideas – **Heal your troubled mind**

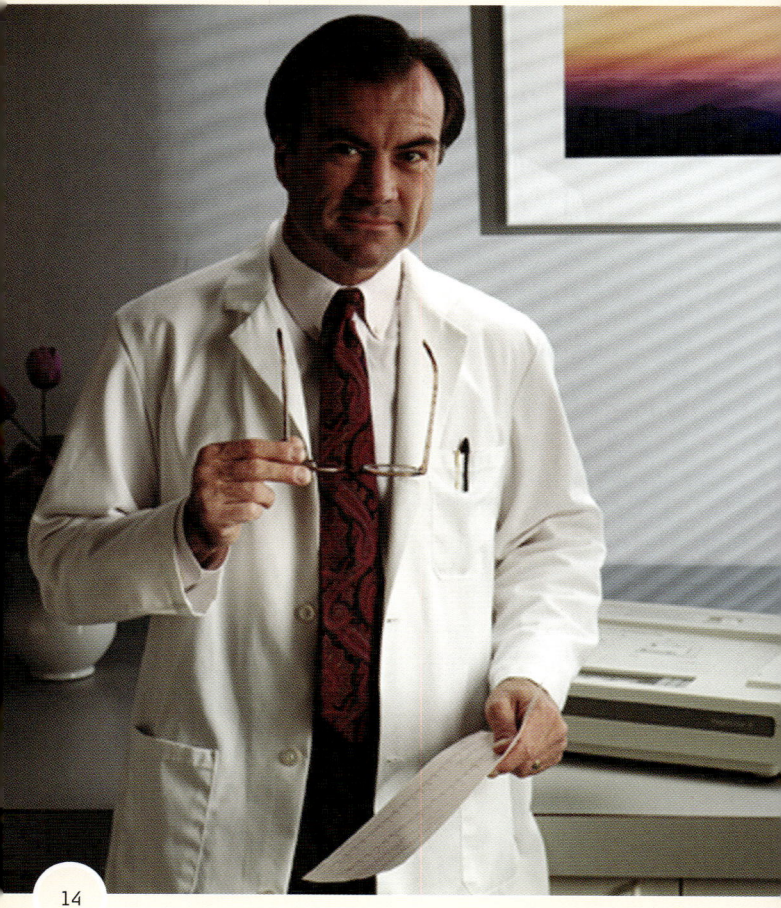

1. Shrinks and quacks

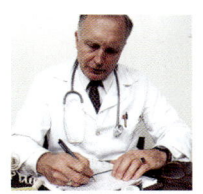

Lots of people claim they'll help you but check out their 'letters' to suss out what they can and can't do for you.

A *psychiatrist* is a doctor, with a degree in medicine and postgraduate training in detecting, diagnosing and treating mental, emotional and behavioural disorders. They are also able to prescribe medication. (Letters to look for: MBBS (medical degree), MD (medical degree in some countries; confusingly it's a postgraduate research degree in others), MRCPsych/FRCPsych (member or fellow of the Royal College of Psychiatrists), MMed Psych, FF Psych, FC Psych (alternatives to MRCPsych in some countries).)

Psychiatric nurses are all-round good guys at the coal face. These are qualified nurses with specialist training, skills and knowledge in treating mental, emotional and behavioural disorders. As well as administering medication, many nurses are trained in one or more talking treatments. The letters to look for are RMN (registered mental nurse).

Psychotherapists use talking to assuage depression and explore feelings and

Defining idea

'He is always saying he is some sort of nerve specialist because it sounds better but everyone knows he is just some sort of janitor in a loony bin.'
P. G. WODEHOUSE

Here's an idea for you...

Your first session should be an assessment. Ask yourself, do I feel confident and at ease seeing this person? Beware of the overwhelmingly glitzy or the underwhelmingly impersonal. Prepare a list of symptoms for the session – feeling morose, sleep problems, loss of appetite or libido, guilt, lethargy etc. It will help plan your treatment.

relationships. By helping you understand the roots of your depression, they guide you towards recovery. You'll usually meet weekly, same time, same place, for fifty minutes. Unfortunately, anyone can call themselves a psychotherapist, but bona-fide ones are members of a professional overseeing body. Don't confuse psychotherapists with *psychoanalysts*. These are the guys with the couches. Up to three times a week, you'll be asked to lie down and talk about your life, relationships, childhood experiences and dreams.

Clinical psychologists have an honours degree in psychology and further postgraduate study. Their job usually involves testing and therapy based on the belief that damaging behaviours can be unlearnt. Psychologists cannot prescribe drugs. (Letters to look for: BSc, PhD.)

There are also *social workers* to help you with issues arising from coping with depression or hospitalisation. They can assist with employment, housing, legal and financial problems. Then there are *occupational therapists,* who are trained professionals using work and leisure activities and relaxation to help you develop or regain skills fundamental to overcoming depression.

2. Run away . . .

. . . or to give it the grown-up name, retreat. Some time alone with your own thoughts is deeply relaxing.

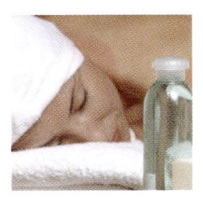

Think just how much noise pollution surrounds us now compared with when we grew up. Televisions in every room; telephones wherever you go; muzak playing where it never played before. This constant barrage is stressful so here are three steps to give yourself a break: 1) switch off the TV, 2) be silent, 3) retreat.

TV will eat up your life. Some nine-year-olds are watching up to four hours a day and these children perform less well on all measures of intelligence and achievement. TV does exactly the same thing to adults. Reclaim hours of your time by limiting TV to one or two favourite programmes a week. The rest of the time, switch it off. Listen to voice radio or music if you must have some noise.

Step 2 is difficult to manage if you live with other people. So take a day off work and experiment with no noise: no TV, radio, no phone – switch it all off. No listening and not talking gives you the chance to hear

Defining idea...

'Silence propagates itself and the longer talk has been suspended, the more difficult it is to find anything to say.'
SAMUEL JOHNSON

Here's an idea for you...

Listen to some Bach, Chopin or Beethoven prior to falling asleep. It's been shown that people who listen to classical music in bed fall asleep more easily and sleep better than people who watch TV or listen to other sorts of music.

what your inner voice is trying to say to you.

For step 3, the best way is to go on a dedicated retreat – all sorts of institutions, religious or otherwise, run them. You can retreat and do yoga or dance or write or paint – or do absolutely nothing. Of course, it's much easier if you can escape but it's not impossible to put aside the hassles of everyday life and retreat in your own home.

Successful retreating at home takes planning. Set aside at least 24 hours, preferably longer. Warn everyone you know that you don't want to be disturbed. Don't open your mail. Don't speak. Limit reading to an hour a day. Do do something creative: write in a journal, paint or draw, invent recipes. This is your opportunity to go inwards and not only relax fully but also work out what you really want to do with your life.

3. Dear diary

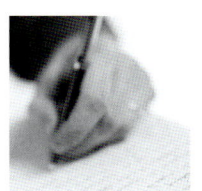

Try some free therapy. Writing a diary can be an oasis of serenity in your life and help you see what really matters.

Keeping a daily diary of important events, thoughts, observations, fears, disappointments, hopes, memories and distress can reduce anxiety, assuage sorrows and help you defeat depression. Over months, your diary will be a great mood barometer, and you'll be able to use it to track your recovery and predict what you need to do to get through future tough times.

In writing things down, you take a step back and that helps you to be much more objective about experiences and how they make you think and feel. After a few weeks you'll start to notice patterns. Some times of the week or parts of your life make you happy and they'll stick out. Once you've realised what they are, doing more of those things is a failsafe remedy. Of course, problems and worries can also seem more real once they're on paper, but this doesn't have to be a bad thing. At least you'll know who the enemy is and what you need to work on.

Defining idea...

'I can shake off everything if I write; my sorrows disappear, my courage is reborn.'
ANNE FRANK

Here's an idea for you...

If you're a dedicated keyboard jockey, why not set up a new email account as your diary, and email your thoughts to this when you have a spare moment at your desk. (Blackberry addicts can even do this on the move.) You can gather the emails together into a proper document at your leisure. What's more, the act of writing to yourself can give a new perspective that you might find useful.

Writing daily gives you a routine and structure, essentials for beating depression. Try to write at the same time of day, as this gets momentum going and wards off inertia in other areas of your life too. You know how your moods vary during the day, so you're well placed to decide when to write. The key is to find a time and place where you can sit comfortably and be relatively uninterrupted.

Getting started is easy. All you need is something to write in (and a pen of course!). That said, those page-per-week appointment diaries just don't cut it. A page per day is the absolute minimum. Why not opt for a loose-leaf binder? You can add pages or cuttings and turn it into a valuable coping resource.

4. Cherish yourself

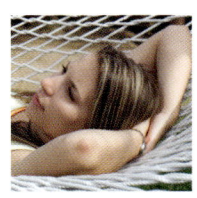

We all know what we ought to do to relax but we often can't be bothered. Start taking relaxation seriously.

Build rock-solid relaxation time into your schedule and treat your appointment to relax as seriously as you do any other. If at all possible, book a professional therapy session once a week. Failing that, schedule time for a DIY treatment at home. Of the various destressing therapies, flotation and reflexology are just two that are effective in lowering the heart rate.

Floating naked in pitch darkness and utter silence for an hour at a time in heavily salted water may sound weird, but you really should try it if you're badly stressed. Sensory deprivation is the closest you can get to experiencing the comfort of the womb. You are all alone with your thoughts but after a while you become disorientated and that's when the magic happens. Some people have almost mystical experiences.

Defining idea...

'There is no need to go to India or anywhere else to find peace. You will find that deep place of silence right in your room, your garden or even your bathtub.'
ELISABETH KUBLER-ROSS, psychiatrist

Here's an idea for you...

Try a quick stretch for instant relaxation. Sit facing a wall. Place your feet on the wall and bring your legs up so that the wall supports them. Edge closer so your backside is only inches from the wall. Lie still and breathe. Support the base of your spine with a cushion if necessary.

Here's the DIY version. Run a bath as deep as you dare and add 500 grams of Dead Sea salts or Epsom salts. Make the bathroom as dark as possible. Set a timer for half an hour. Then soak in the bath. (Don't do this if you are pregnant or have a medical condition.) Go straight to bed afterwards – and be careful: you may feel light-headed. When you wake, have a warm shower.

Reflexology is an ancient treatment and it's far more sophisticated than a mere foot rub. Having your feet cradled and massaged grounds you and is instantly calming. The theory is that all nerves originate in the spine and branch out through the body but ultimately all connect with the nerves that end in the foot. Each area of the foot therefore corresponds to an area of the body.

Here's the DIY version. First relax your feet in a footbath of tepid water and a few drops of peppermint oil. Then massage your feet using your thumb to make small circling movements over the whole sole of each foot. When you find a tender spot, work on it gently – this indicates an area where you have tension.

5. Listen up

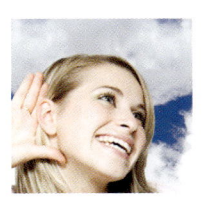

The right music can move you from brow beaten to bouncy in just three minutes. Find your pearls of pop Prozac.

As filmmakers, advertisers and Mr Whippy sellers know, playing the right tune can put you in the mood for love, new trainers or a cornet with a flake. But music can also help your troubled mind. Music therapy is a powerful psychological treatment that uses instrumental and vocal activities to change moods, explore feelings, promote self-expression and increase self-esteem. Ten years ago, researchers at Stanford Medical School studied three groups of patients. The first group received a weekly visit from a music therapist, the second group used music therapy techniques but didn't see a therapist, and the third group didn't have any form of musical intervention. People in the first two groups had significantly better mood and raised self-esteem and these benefits lasted.

To reap some benefits from music therapy, you don't need to see a therapist. Chances are, you can start to heal your mind with whatever's in your CD collection. Go for whatever strikes a chord and suits how you're

Defining idea...

'Why waste money on psychotherapy when you can listen to Bach's B Minor Mass?'
MICHAEL TORKE, composer

Here's an idea for you...

Make a compilation tape or download tracks to make a personalised mood-busting playlist for your MP3 player. That way, whether you're into Motown or mountain dulcimer, you'll always have music to move you when you need a boost.

feeling. For instance, if you're having another duvet day with Enya, you might need to switch to Eminem. Music that's fast and furious wakes up your body and brain. Anything that makes you move is perfect.

Sometimes when you're feeling low, it helps to listen to slow sentimental mush and have a good cry. Many pros believe that the way to go is to start with music that matches your mood and then move on to more happy, upbeat sounds. If you're feeling anxious, music with a slow beat will slow your breathing and racing pulse. Gentle compositions help release muscle tension and lower blood pressure. Choose music with a slow rhythm, ideally slower than your heart rate, which will be about 70 beats per minute.

Next time you're feeling stressed, take a 'sound bath'. Put some music on your sound system, then cosy up close to the speakers. As you listen, imagine the sound washing over you, rinsing off your stress. Listen in the dark or with your eyes closed, as your hearing will sharpen when you can't see.

Idea 6 – **Aromatherapy?!**

6. Aromatherapy?!

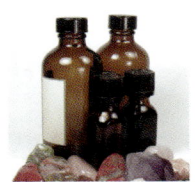

Yes, aromatherapy kicks ass, and it works. Try it for yourself – the proof of the pudding is in the eating.

Here's a challenge. Next time you're writing your 'to-do' list, put 'Do something lovely for me' at the top of the list and give it top priority. If you're laughing at the very thought of such self-indulgence, then you need this idea because it works – fast. Many people see aromatherapy as a bit of a joke. How often have you read 'sprinkle a little lavender oil in your bath to destress you'? How often have you wondered how you'll find the time for a shower, much less a bath? Let's face it, the people who can find the time to do the lavender oil stuff probably don't have too much stress in the first place.

If you're in that camp, you should listen to Judith White, an inspirational aromatherapist who believes aromatherapy can do a lot more than make your bath smell nice. 'Aromatherapy is perfect for those times when you have only seconds because it works in seconds and it is one of the most valuable tools we have to help us live a less

Defining idea...

'Smell is a potent wizard that transports you across thousands of miles and all the years you have lived.'
HELEN KELLER

Here's an idea for you...

Build up an 'armoury' of oils. Lavender is great when you need to calm down or drift off to sleep. Cedarwood is good when you're anxious or stressed. Geranium is good for making you feel in control. Grapefruit or *may chang* for when you're feeling low. Clary sage when you're feeling paranoid or oversensitive (but, alas, avoid this if you're pregnant), and *ylang ylang* when you want to boost your self-esteem and feel confident and sensual.

stressed life,' she says. She speaks from personal experience. 'I had to learn how to maintain my equilibrium when I was emotionally, mentally and physically stressed for an extremely difficult few years. My oils were my greatest ally.'

She recommends you look for opportunities throughout your day to stick in a mini-multi-tasking treatment. Oils aren't just for baths. When showering, cover the plughole with a flannel and add 4–6 drops (in total) of a combination of essential oils to the shower tray. Add one drop of essential oil to your existing moisturiser. Inhale deeply as you apply it. Try soaking your feet in an aromatic footbath whilst reading or watching TV. For an immediate treatment put a couple of drops of essential oil into the middle of a hot, wet flannel, wring it out, hold it over your face and breath deeply

7. Beat those blues

A little bit of what you fancy does you good so build some enjoyment into every day.

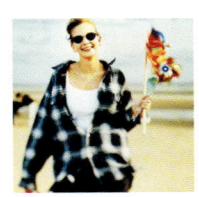

Depression saps energy and motivation. You're tired, you feel flat, fed up and life just isn't fun anymore. Hardly surprising you don't feel like doing anything. Have you stopped going out with friends, dropped out of paragliding or left your bike rusting in the shed for a second consecutive Christmas? Is it such a big deal? Frankly, yes, because once you've given up enjoyable activities, you'll start a cycle that'll make you feel worse and you'll end up doing even less.

It's time to puncture your vicious cycle of inactivity. How? Think of the kind of stuff that used to make your heart soar. No matter if it was kickboxing, karaoke or knitting, it's time to do it again. When we do things we love, we forget ourselves, lose track of time and dismal thoughts take a back seat. Doing just one thing that's fun or that gives you that warm glow of achievement will make you feel better. In fact, even planning to do something you enjoy can cause a mini buzz.

Defining idea...

'Happiness consists in activity. It is a running stream, not a stagnant pool.'
JOHN MASON GOOD, physician and author

Here's an idea for you...

Mulling over enjoyable times can also hike up your mood. Start a journal or photo diary to look at when your mood is especially low and use it to spur you on when you feel like staying in bed.

Doing what you enjoy has what pros call a 'dose-response effect'. This means that the more you do, the better you'll feel. It doesn't have to bust your budget or take all afternoon. Here are some simple ideas to lift black moods: phone a friend, take a yoga class or have a massage, watch a big match or a funny film, plant a shrub, dance to a CD. Be realistic about what you're going to do, though: three rows of knitting before lunch, rather than three stripy jumpers with matching bobble hats.

Some people feel guilty about doing fun things when there's a pile of ironing to be done, mouths to feed, reports to write and deadlines loom. However, what they don't realise is doing things that are entertaining or exciting helps us do more of those essentials. Once you've got your head around this, you'll stop feeling guilty about taking time out for yourself.

8. Perfect moments

If you develop the skill to create perfect moments, you'll guarantee that tomorrow will be less stressed than today.

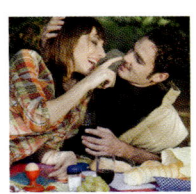

For the most part, the formula for happiness is quite simple. Happy people don't get so busy stressing about building a 'perfect' tomorrow that they forget to enjoy this 'perfect' today. It turns out that the surest, indeed, the only predictor of how happy you are going to be in the future is how good you are at being happy today. If you want to know if you are going to be stressed out tomorrow, ask yourself what are you doing to diminish your stress today. And if the answer's 'nothing', you won't be that calm and serene person you long to be any time soon.

We can plan the perfect party, perfect marriage, perfect career etc but we have absolutely no idea if when we get 'there', a perfect 'anything' is going to deliver. The only thing we can do is guarantee that today at least we will have a perfect moment – a moment of no stress where we pursue pure joy.

Defining idea...

'Happiness not in another place, but this place, not in another hour, but this hour.'
WALT WHITMAN

Here's an idea for you...

Invest in an old-fashioned teasmade. Waking up to a cup of tea in bed can get the day off to a good start for little effort on your part.

Your perfect moment might be snatched late at night, listening to jazz by candlelight when the family are asleep. Or it could be a glass of chilled wine as the sun slips beyond the horizon. You might best be able to access a perfect moment by running round your park or through practising yoga. Preparing, cooking and eating food can give perfect moments. Gardening is a good one. Sex is reliable. All you have to do is give yourself the space to feel it more often – ideally, at least once a day.

Ultimately, only you know your own triggers. Write down a week's worth and plan for them. Schedule them in your diary. It obviously doesn't have to be the same activity every day and sometimes despite your best intentions, it all goes belly up. But planning for perfect moments means they are more likely to happen. Even if you don't believe now that striving for perfect moments will destress you, try it. At least you will be able to say 'Today, there were five minutes where I stopped and enjoyed life.' Enjoying life today is the only certainty you have of happiness and your best chance of being less stressed tomorrow.

9. It's your time

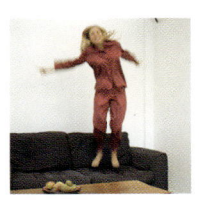

When you're feeling crushed by your things-to-do list, good time management can transform your mood and your life.

Concentration problems are rife in depression, but a to-do list means you won't forget that hairdresser's appointment or leave your washing in the machine overnight. And nothing really beats the sense of achievement you get from putting another tick by a task. Using 'to-do' lists decreases stress, develops great organisational skills and improves your memory. Just writing things down means you are 25% more likely to do them. Go one better with a daily list that'll show you at a glance what you need to prioritise and what can wait. One method is the ABC list. This list is divided into three sections: A (do today), B (do this week) and C (do this month). As the B or C items become more pertinent they can be bumped up to the A or B list.

Get to know your body clock and exploit it. If you're freshest in the early morning, use that time to do difficult tasks, like writing a letter to your bank manager about that unauthorised overdraft. Mechanical

Defining idea...

'Time equals life. Therefore, waste your time and waste your life, or master your time and master your life.'

ALAN LAKEIN, time management guru

Here's an idea for you...

If you're seeing a therapist or doctor, ask for the first appointment of the day or first appointment after their lunch break. That'll mean you won't waste time in the waiting room because they're running late.

jobs like loading the washing machine can be left for when you're feeling brain dead and worn out.

If you're sluggish in the mornings, you can sneak up to fifteen minutes extra in bed by a bit of planning the night before. Put cereal (minus milk) into a bowl, fill the kettle and put out a mug. Get the next day's clothes ready. There's very little worse than getting up and needing to iron a clean shirt.

You probably wouldn't eat a family-size bar of chocolate in one go – you'd break it into smaller chunks. Do the same with the massive jobs on your list. For instance, if you're feeling too low and weary to fill in another job application form, chunk it up and start with the easy questions you don't need to think about, like your name, address and date of birth. Once you've got some momentum going, add in things that need more concentration, like your job history.

Idea 10 – **Don't act on impulse**

10. Don't act on impulse

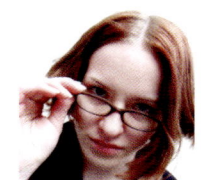

Focus, concentrate: stick to what you've started. That will cut your stress levels instantly.

When you get to bed, do you remember the stuff that you didn't get round to and feel disappointed and frustrated with yourself? When that happens it's time to go back to basics and use this idea. It helps you finish what you start and makes you feel on top of your life. Besides helping you become more focused, it also helps you curb your impulse to wander off and do other stuff rather than the one task that you have set yourself.

Before you go to bed tonight, think of something you want to achieve tomorrow. Keep it really small and simple – for example cleaning the cutlery drawer. It doesn't matter what it is, but you have to do it. Take it extremely seriously: *promise* yourself you'll do it – and follow through.

Here's an idea for you...

Every time you keep a promise to yourself, stick some loose change in a jar. It's a good visual record of your growing focus and strength – and, of course, you get to spend the cash at the end of it.

If you make a promise to yourself every evening for a week, and follow through, you can take the next step by listing some tasks that you need to undertake but have been putting off. Break down any big tasks into manageable chunks. You will need at least seven. Each night for the next week, pick one thing from the list and promise yourself you'll do it tomorrow. Keep that promise. Don't let impulse drive you off course.

This is an exercise in mental toughness. Making promises to yourself that you never keep brings you down and, over time, breaks your heart. But by breaking difficult tasks down into manageable chunks and building the strength of character to follow through and get them out of the way, you take a huge step forward in reducing stress in your life. It will also build your self-esteem and clear your life of a ton of irritations that have been stopping you mentally from moving on.

Defining idea...

'He who every morning plans the transactions of the day and follows out that plan, carries a thread that will guide him through the maze of the most busy life. But when no plan is laid, when the disposal of time is surrendered merely to the chance of coincidence, chaos will soon reign.'
VICTOR HUGO

Idea 11 – **Counting sheep**

11. Counting sheep

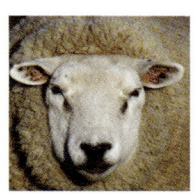

Quality sleep is a serious depression buster. Here are some reliable routes to regular, refreshing rest.

Some disruption of sleep is due to messed up brain chemicals, but worries that accompany stress and depression often prevent us relaxing sufficiently to fall asleep. Sleeping pills are addictive and often leave people feeling hungover the next day. They're almost always a bad idea. So, what else can we do?

It can help to have evening routines that give bodies and minds a chance to wind down – some light reading, soothing music or a warm bath. Another, good tactic is only going to bed if you're tired. If you're not asleep after thirty minutes, get up and only go back to bed when you're sleepy. Losing a bit of sleep won't hurt.

Where chemical help is concerned, melatonin is a supplement that helps some people with insomnia. Our bodies make melatonin, releasing it in increasing amounts from dusk. If you decide to top yours up, give it a

Defining idea...

'Sleep is when all the unsorted stuff comes flying out as from a dustbin upset in a high wind.'
WILLIAM GOLDING

Here's an idea for you...

Once you've set your alarm clock, put it out of sight and avoid checking it if you wake up in the night. Clockwatching can cause insomnia.

couple of weeks to see any difference. Valerian is a herbal medicine that some people find helpful.

Tea, coffee, cigarettes and even that innocent-looking cup of cocoa are stimulants. It's worth cutting these out for two weeks to see if they're culpable. Perhaps you've found that a stiff drink helps you fall asleep, but are puzzled why you don't feel rested the next day. Alcohol messes up our natural sleep rhythms. When you have a large whisky, you're giving yourself the equivalent of a general anaesthetic. You miss out on the type of sleep you need for that refreshed feeling.

Falling asleep too early? In the evenings, sit near a bright light to reset your body clock. When it's time for bed, keep your bedroom dark. And how hot is your bedroom? Most of us sleep better in a cool room, so try leaving a window open or turning down your central heating.

If all else fails, count sheep. Visualise them clambering over a gate, one by one. As you start to drop off, your mind might wander and you'll lose count. Never mind, just start again. The monotony is more important than whether any sheep made a break for it when you weren't looking.

12. Out to get you

Are you ready for a journey to the weirder, wilder side? Relax. We're only talking a little white witchery.

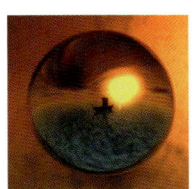

Here's the truth – sometimes the bastards *are* out to get you. We know all the arguments about wishing well to the world, good karma, turning the other cheek. We may practise all of them. But sometimes, through no fault of your own, you become the scapegoat – the victim in life.

Human beings have a very powerful need for scapegoats. No one gets through life without feeling they're being picked on at some time. Money doesn't protect you from it; power doesn't protect you from it. It's incredibly hard to accept that, despite your competence and general sweetness of personality, other people don't wish you well. Just remember other people have their own agenda and you don't always know what that is. So what do you do?

You build up psychic defence. 'One of the major reasons we feel attacked or got at,' writes Caitlin Matthews, 'is that we become neglectful of our boundaries, not noticing when

Defining idea...

'Psychic protection is an ordinary skill for everyday life.'
CAITLIN MATTHEWS, author of *The Psychic Protection Handbook*

Here's an idea for you...

When you're feeling stressed and under attack, immerse yourself in mechanical repetitive tasks. Cooking works well; so does weeding the garden. Concentrate fully on your actions. Switch off your brain. You'll soon feel more centred.

someone or something is taking advantage of us.' Reflect on where your boundaries are weak and strengthen those areas.

A good way of grounding yourself is by exercising. Bring your mind back to your body as often as you remember and note what you are feeling. If you're tired, sleep. Eat and drink warm and comforting food. Be in nature. There is great comfort in looking after the basics.

To deal with bad karma, build a shield around you. Sit quietly and find your still centre and then imagine a bubble of gold, silver or rosy pink enclosing your body and the energy field that surrounds your body – which you are more likely to be conscious of as your 'personal space'. Throughout the day remind yourself it's there and see the outside of this shield sparkling and fizzing with energy. Cover yourself in this imaginary psychic armour. Breathe out your fear; breathe in courage. Say aloud, 'I am protected. No harm will I give; no harm will I receive.' Remember to be grateful for the protection.

13. Drop if you stop?

If the lurgy blights the first week of your holiday, that's leisure sickness – 'stop and collapse' syndrome.

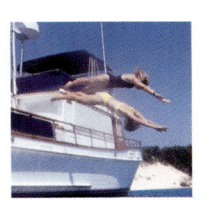

Those who suffer with 'stop and collapse syndrome' share certain characteristics: a high workload, perfectionism, eagerness to achieve, and an overdeveloped sense of responsibility to their work – all of which makes it difficult to switch off.

One theory is that those who work hard simply get so bored on holiday that they start to notice the symptoms they've been suppressing while at work. It could also be a case of 'mind over matter': we don't allow ourselves to get sick until the work is done. Yet another theory is that when you're working (stressed) your immune system is actually working better than it does when you're relaxing. When you relax, so does your immune system, and kaboom, you're calling the concierge for a doctor. So, what can you do about it?

For a start, you should support your local immune system. Eat a minimum of five portions of fruit and veg a day and take a good-quality

Defining idea...

'Those who don't take the time to be well eventually have to find the time to be ill.'
Anon.

Here's an idea for you...

If you're prone to weekend sickness, try exercising on Friday evenings. Exercise is a stressor but one your body loves. This acts as a transition between work and time off, and helps you unwind quicker.

multivitamin and mineral supplement (e.g. Bioforce, Solgar, Viridian, Vitabiotics). If you drink too much alcohol or are a smoker, you also need more vitamin C – so supplement that too. Echinacea can also be good, so give it a try as well (but read the instructions carefully).

Plan for holidays with military precision. Assuming that you've checked your passports will be valid at the time of your holiday, you really need to start gradually winding down two to three weeks before you go.

Three weeks before departure, make a packing list. Write down everything you need to take with you and then allocate each lunchtime that week to completing any associated errands. Two weeks before you go, sort out work. Take a look at all your projects and decide at what stage you want to freeze or pass them over. Set goals with each project and allocate deadlines for reaching them preferably all to be tied up the day before your last day.

One week before departure, start packing. Put out your bags or suitcases in a spare room if you've got one and start the washing and ironing nightmare. Do a little packing each night. Before you know it, you'll be ready to go.

Idea 13 – **Drop if you stop?**

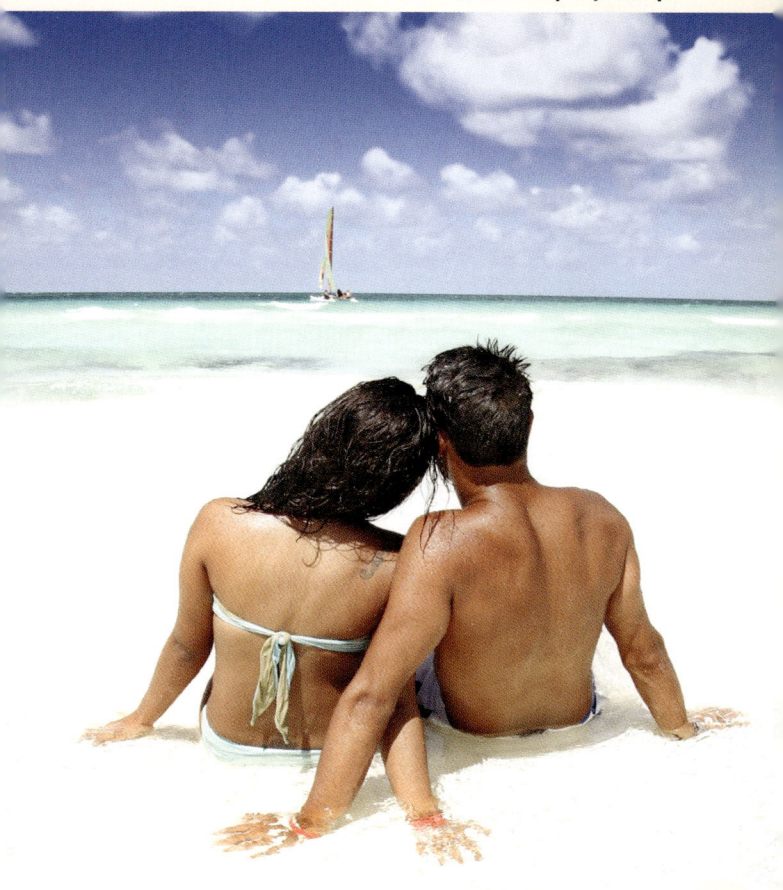

52 Brilliant Ideas – **Heal your troubled mind**

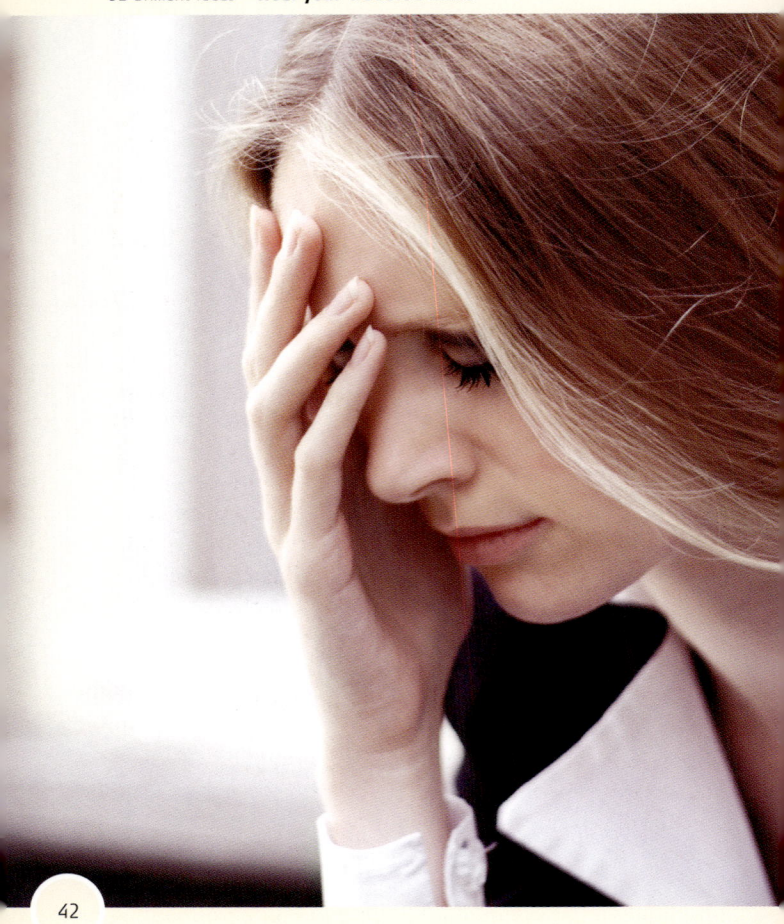

14. Feeling SAD?

For many people, less daylight equals less happiness. Use these illuminating tips to avoid another winter of discontent.

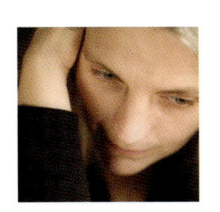

Sun shortage can cause sadness ranging from dark moods to a condition called seasonal affective disorder or SAD. A diagnosis of SAD can only be made after three or more consecutive winters of symptoms. SAD symptoms are similar to non-seasonal depression but rather than losing weight or waking early, if you've got SAD you're more likely to oversleep and reach for the biscuit jar to satisfy carb cravings.

In northern Sweden there are only a few hours of winter daylight and some days with no light at all. Psychiatrists there, working with depressed patients, demonstrated the benefits of light boxes in treating SAD. If you plump for a light box, use it daily from when your first symptoms appear. You'll need to sit an arm's length away for between 60 to 90 minutes. You don't have to put your life on hold: you can read, work, eat – do anything you like as long as you're reasonably stationary. Many people feel better after three or four days but that wears off unless it's used every day.

Defining idea...

'How heavy the days are. There is not a fire that can warm me, nor a sun to laugh with me.'
HERMAN HESSE, Steppenwolf

Here's an idea for you...

Plan a 'summer' holiday in winter. A couple of weeks of long daylight hours to tide you over until spring may be just what the doctor ordered. Why just dream of a white (sandy beach) Christmas?

Vitamin D deficiency plays a role in SAD. No great surprise, as it's been called the sunshine vitamin. Ultraviolet rays from sunlight react in your skin, producing a form of vitamin D. People with SAD who took a 400 IU vitamin D supplement (equivalent to a teaspoon of cod liver oil) every day for five days noticed a lift in their winter blues.

Nobody likes the taste of cod liver oil, so you might like to try prawns, sardines, mackerel or salmon instead – these foods are rich in vitamin D. If you're a vegetarian you'll get small amounts of vitamin D from creamy milk and egg yolks. If you're vegan, you'll need to eat fortified foods, like soy milk, margarine and breakfast cereal, and take vitamin D supplements.

And if you're prone to the winter blues, try to make the most out of what sunshine there is. Wrap up warm and enjoy a good walk: your vitamin D levels will thank you for it.

15. Your dark side

Reckon you're not an angry person? Maybe that's why you're so stressed.

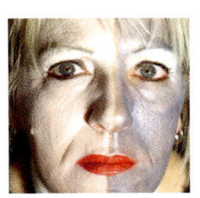

Displaced anger isn't so much a problem with some people, as a vocation. An awful lot of us displace our anger into other emotions. That's because we don't like anger in our culture. The reason we don't like it is that we're never taught how to acknowledge it, deal with it, use it – and that leads to mucho stress.

Why does suppressing anger make us stressed? According to psychiatrist Theodore Rubin, people attempt to feel only those feelings that fit in with their view of themselves. But, by suppressing their 'dark side', they put their emotions in a deep freeze, lose their capacity to feel all emotions as acutely and run the risk of living half a life.

Anger is as valid as any other emotion, says Theodore. And it's one we suffer from a lot. Psychiatrists believe we get angry every time we're hurt or let down, but those of us for whom anger is a no-no learn to

Defining idea...

'Depression is nothing but anger without enthusiasm.'
STEVEN WRIGHT, comedian

Here's an idea for you...

When you're upset, go to a quiet place and have a good groan. Big theatrical groans really help to dissipate stress.

pervert the anger into another emotion and it becomes anxiety, bitterness or depression.

At anger workshops, you can 'find' your anger. The leader of one such workshop tells us that anger has to be expressed both physically and verbally. She stands in front of a large beanbag (it could have been a bed or a pile of pillows) and whacks the hell out of it with a plastic baseball bat. 'Focus on the person you're angry with,' she says calmly. 'Imagine they are the beanbag.' Scary, perhaps, but then the anger is out and nobody gets hurt.

The idea is to thump and bellow your rage on the down swing. It takes practice. If you find it hard to find your voice, just concentrate on developing a rhythm. Let the feelings come in their own time. And they will. If you do this when you're angry, you'll defuse stress in a matter of minutes. You won't be such a nice person, but life will be a lot more straightforward. Once you start bashing out your anger, life gets a lot more fun.

16. All in the mind

Ever wondered what's happening in your brain when you get depressed? This idea explains brain science.

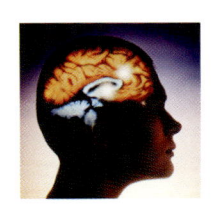

When we're depressed, our brains work differently.

Your brain is a colony of ten billion cells that communicate with each other. Between each cell there are spaces called synapses. A synapse is a sort of junction between two brain cells, where the end of one almost touches another. Electrical charges are used to communicate inside brain cells but the electricity doesn't carry across the synapse. Instead, brain cells release chemical communicators. These chemical communicators are usually stored in little capsules called vesicles and, when needed, swim into synapses, carrying their message to the next cell ensuring communication carries on uninterrupted.

These chemical communicators are called neurotransmitters. Nobody knows for sure how many neurotransmitters there are, but at the last count there were over forty. They carry different messages. Some get their part of the brain turned on and excited,

Defining idea...

'Men ought to know that from nothing else but the brain come joys, delights, laughter, grief, despondency and lamentations.'
HIPPOCRATES

Here's an idea for you...

Ask your physician or pharmacist to explain how your drugs work. A basic knowledge of brain chemistry will wow these pros and encourage them to explain properly what's going on. There's no need to be fobbed off with some cruddy explanation.

others put a damper on things. Here's the lowdown on two of them.

Serotonin drives our sleep and wake cycles. You might have heard that levels of serotonin are lower in people with depression. Instead of spreading communication in the synapse between adjacent brain cells, serotonin is reabsorbed, so communications about mood, sleep, appetite and sex drive are lost.

Noradrenaline is like a party planner, controlling brain activity. But when you're depressed, noradrenaline is released from brain cells at a snail's pace, so activity levels plummet.

Brain cells are covered in receptors for these chemical communicators. In the same way that your house key only fits one front door in your street, receptors are shaped so that only one type of neurotransmitter will fit.

Your brain is a great recycler. Once neurotransmitters have done their thing, the brain cell that fired them out takes them back in. This is called reuptake. Many antidepressants work by stopping reuptake. Selective serotonin reuptake inhibitors (SSRIs), for example, prevent serotonin from being recycled, so there's more of it around, allowing those important brain signals to complete their journey.

17. Learn to bounce

Everyone gets stressed but some people are better at dealing with it than others. That's because they're natural 'bouncers'.

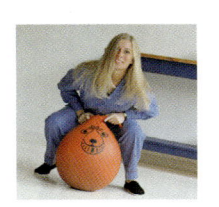

Disappointment does one of two things: it makes you 'bouncy' (resilient) or it makes you 'bitter' – and which way you respond is a telling predictor of future happiness. Bounce-ability is easy for idealistic twenty-somethings. But during our thirties, the decisions we make pretty well determine what sort of person we're going to be, and how we decide to deal with setbacks is one of the greatest determinants.

According to psychologist Dr Al Siebert, bouncers exhibit flexibility. 'If you look at someone who doesn't handle life well,' he writes, 'it's often because they think, feel or act in only one way and can't see any alternative.' That means they get stuck in an idea of the sort of person they have to be, the sort of job they were meant to do, the sort of partner that's right for them, the sort of life that they 'deserve'.

Defining idea...

'Hope begins in the dark. The stubborn hope that if you just show up and try to do the right thing the dawn will come. You wait and watch and work. You don't give up.'
ANNE LAMOTT, writer

Here's an idea for you...

Next time you're in the middle of a crisis, try to laugh every chance you can. And if you can't laugh, cry. One way or another, vent your emotions. Your mind will work better when strong feelings aren't interfering with your ability to think straight.

Each of us is born, apparently, with a happiness set-point, which is genetically influenced but, crucially, not fixed. Remember this: your brain chemistry is not fixed. You can change it.

How? Well, when bad stuff happens, ask yourself what are known as 'coping questions' that challenge inflexible thinking. What is the reality, and what is merely my fantasy about this situation? Can I salvage anything from this? Then ask yourself some 'serendipity questions'. Why is it good that this has happened? What am I learning from this? What could I do to turn this situation around?

Ultimately, what it comes down to is remembering that everything changes and change itself is the source of stress. Bad stuff happens to good people. But there are plenty of people who have had every disappointment in the book and still lived useful, happy lives. And science will tell you that there's no reason why you can't be one of the bouncers too.

18. Go on, prove it

New miracle cures grace every health page, but which ones works? Here's a guide to help you sort fact from hype.

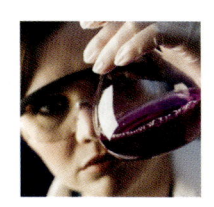

Sangam yoga and green tea enemas may be the tabloid treatment of the week, but how do you know which claims to take at face value? It can be hard to know what to trust. There have always been quacks and charlatans tricking the vulnerable with 'miracle' cures. But it's also true that many well-meaning people publish information on defeating depression that's confusing, unhelpful or biased, so you need to be at least one step ahead of them. How? Look at scientific research using key principles from evidence-based medicine.

Evidence-based medicine, according to its originator, Professor Dave Sackett, is 'conscientious, explicit and judicious use of current best evidence in making decisions about the care of individual patients'. Critics dismiss it as a new-fangled fad, but its roots go back to the mid-nineteenth century.

Next time you hear or read about a new treatment, be sceptical. First ask, *what's this claim based on?* There's a pecking order for looking at research

Defining idea...

'Show me the money!'
JERRY MAGUIRE, the movie

Here's an idea for you...

Buy a medical dictionary and read up on the science behind the treatments you've been offered or are considering. The *BMJ* and *Lancet* are accessible medical journals for the lay-person and many journals are now online. Befriend a librarian first to learn how to search scientific literature online and how to access information.

studies, as some are superior to others. The top two types of research papers are called meta-analyses and randomised controlled trials. In meta-analysis researchers collect studies and comb through them, combining results from only the high-quality research. Randomised controlled trials are studies that find out if a treatment works. Researchers compare the effects of having the new treatment against having an inactive treatment.

If it is a randomised controlled trial, ask *is this control group fair and relevant?* If one group has three green tea enemas a week, while the other group gets a five-minute phone call, the enema group might be getting better because they are having extra attention and human contact, rather than green tea. On the other hand, if the control group have caffeine enemas rather than phone calls and didn't get better, then there might be something in it.

Who paid for it? If research into sangam yoga is funded by the National Sangam Yoga Society, they've probably got vested interest. Big bucks can lead to invalid support for preconceived notions or unfairly influence scientists or publishers.

19. Turning Japanese

Learn from Zen. The Japanese bath and tea ceremonies were as much about refreshing the spirit as cleansing the body.

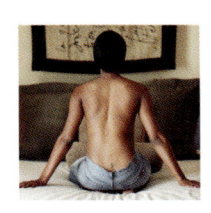

Try out the ceremony of the Japanese bath and you'll see why the Japanese consider having a bath to be a sacred experience. Make time for this once a week. It's a better stress-buster than a simple candle-lit bath, perhaps because you have to put a tad of extra effort in and that makes us feel we're taking back control.

First, light an aromatherapy burner in the bathroom, lock the door and sit there quietly breathing in the fragrance, letting your mind quieten and be still. Keep your focus on what you can see, feel, hear and smell. Let go of all other thoughts. If anxious thoughts intrude, imagine them drifting off in the fragrance rising from the burner. When you're relaxed, undress and gently draw a brush or loofah over your body, working always towards the heart. Then step into the shower – lather up and get really clean. Concentrate on the noise of the shower.

Defining idea...

'There must be quite a few things a hot bath won't cure, but I don't know any of them.'
SYLVIA PLATH

Here's an idea for you...

Invest in some special props that you keep purely for your bath. The sense of 'specialness' helps turn it into an event and with time you will be able to trigger relaxation with just part of the ritual. A cup of tea, a bath with the balancing oil or body brushing will in themselves be almost as good as the whole ritual.

Clean? Now step out the shower and sink into a hot bath containing a few drops of your favourite balancing oil. When intrusive worrying thoughts interrupt, let them gently float away in the steam. Use a small bowl to ladle water all over your body and focus your mind on pouring the water as gracefully as possible. Let yourself enter a sort of trance state, soothed by the repetitive actions.

When your mind is calm and you feel centred, emerge and wrap yourself in a warm dressing gown. Then light candles and make some tea, concentrating fully on every step. Make your movements as graceful and economical as possible. Green tea gives the authentic 'Eastern' feeling, but any tea will do. Finally, retire to a quiet, cosy place, sip your tea, inhale the fragrance, focus on the candle flames. Imagine anxious thoughts drifting away in the fragrant steam rising from your cup.

20. Magnetic attraction

Can magnets max your mood? Well, believe it or not, transcranial magnetic therapy has a lot going for it.

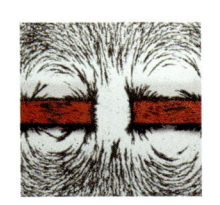

Chinese medical practitioners have used magnetic treatments for depression for the last two millennia, and some Tibetan monks alleviate depression using magnetic forces. Trials over here with a pioneering treatment using magnets have shown promise.

Patients with severe, life-threatening depression are sometimes treated with electroconvulsive therapy (ECT). ECT is the most powerful antidepressant we've got, and, unlike drugs, it works instantly, which can literally be life-saving for people who are so depressed they have stopped eating and drinking. It has its fans, but also harsh critics because of the lasting memory problems it can cause. During ECT, electricity is fired through the brain, causing uncontrolled brain activity, resulting in a fit. Transcranial magnetic therapy (TMS) distributes its get-up-and-go in a more controlled way. Unlike ECT, you don't need an anaesthetic and it

Defining idea...

Stars open among the lilies. Are you not blinded by such expressionless sirens? This is the silence of astounded souls.
SYLVIA PLATH

Here's an idea for you...

You may be able to try transcranial magnetic therapy by taking part in a trial. Why not ask your doctor if this is being offered locally?

doesn't jumble your memory. Being awake means you can chat or read during treatment. This new procedure is useful for drug-resistant severe depression.

During treatment, you wear a funky cloth hat that looks like a bathing cap, but with lines drawn on it so your doctor can see exactly where to place and hold the magnet. A powerful magnetic coil is then held over a place at the front of your head called the left dorsolateral prefrontal cortex – it's just behind your forehead. Big judgements, planning and decisions get made there. There's strong evidence suggesting that the left prefrontal cortex is underactive in depression. Many people think TMS works by heightening this activity.

As the doctor holds the magnet, a number of painless magnetic pulses pass through your skull. This process makes a noise a bit like a pecking woodpecker. These pulses induce electric currents, altering and aiding brain activity. Each treatment lasts around twenty minutes. Unfortunately, you'll need a course of treatment: usually two or three days a week for a fortnight.

TMS could be a good alternative to ECT, but some people remain to be convinced. Preliminary results from trials on real people with real depression are promising, but it could still be some time before it's available at a clinic near you.

21. Crisis management

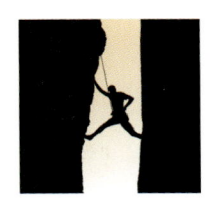

Facing the week from hell? This is the toolbox for navigating through those really stressful, busy times.

We've all been there. On really busy days, with deadlines looming, we get to the stage where we're scared to answer the phone in case it's someone demanding something else. So it's time to decide to stop being such a victim. Why fear the worst until it happens? Every time a negative thought crosses your brain, cancel it out with a positive one.

Develop a mantra to suit whatever crisis you're in today, something you can say to yourself mindlessly every time your mind goes into tailspin. For instance, when the panic hits, chant 'I am serenely gliding towards my deadline and everything will get done'. Do it enough to believe it, and you'll feel much better.

The 'best use' question is invaluable in negotiating your way through any day with dozens of calls on your time. It helps you to prioritise 'on

Defining idea...

'There cannot be a crisis next week. My schedule is already full.'
HENRY KISSINGER

Here's an idea for you...

Keep a time log of your working week so you finally get a realistic idea of how long it takes you to complete all your usual activities. This means you stop kidding yourself about how quickly you will perform tasks in an imperfect world – where you're interrupted frequently – and you'll reduce your stress levels hugely.

the run', sometimes quite ruthlessly. Each morning, decide what you've got to achieve that day and if anything interrupts, ask yourself 'Is this the best use of my time, right now?' If the answer's 'no', take a raincheck. So if a friend calls you at work, don't chat then – unless it's a genuine emergency – say you'll call back. Likewise, don't let colleagues sidetrack you with petty queries or complaints.

A lot of stress is of our own making. One of the biggest mistakes is to tell people what they want to hear without thinking if it's feasible for you. If you promise results you can't deliver without a lot of stress, you've shot yourself in the foot. Aim at under-promising rather than over-promising. That way your friends are delighted when you turn up at the party you said you couldn't make and your boss thinks you're wonderful when you get the report finished a day early rather than a week late. Make it your rule from now on to be absolutely realistic about how long it's going to take you to get things done. Until you get expert at this, work out the time you reckon it will take you to complete any task and multiply it by 1.5.

22. Get the cream

Wanna feel like the CAT that got the cream? You're just sixteen weeks from happiness with cognitive analytic therapy.

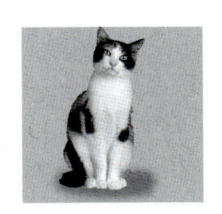

Cognitive analytic therapy (CAT) is a no-nonsense therapy developed as a way to treat people suffering depression in a short time. Most people have sixteen sessions, but you may need as few as four. What's in the name? Cognitive means using your thoughts about yourself. Analytic means getting down to the nitty-gritty of the forces that drive what you do. Therapy means helping you defeat depression through increased self-awareness. In CAT, you'll work with a therapist to look at what has slowed down or stalled positive changes in your past. Unlike other talking treatments, CAT puts the spotlight on how problems develop and shows you what's wrong with your ways of coping with bad times. What makes this therapy a winner is that it's adapted to your life. Your strong points are the power for change.

You'll be asked to tell your story so the therapist will start to understand more about your life and what makes you tick. After about four sessions,

Defining idea...

'Cognitive analytic therapy occupies the centre ground as the New Labour of talking treatments: tough on the problem, tough on the causes of the problem.'
DR PAUL BLENKIRON, psychiatrist

Here's an idea for you...

Start a diary of your moods and actions. It'll be a great help when you go for an assessment with a therapist. Keeping a diary while waiting for therapy may mean you get even more out of cognitive analytic therapy and it could shorten your treatment.

you'll be given a 'reformulation letter' describing your life so far, difficulties you've struggled with and how you've survived them, and some new ways of seeing your problems. You'll have plenty of time to think about these observations and make factual changes. You'll either learn something about yourself you didn't know before, or see something you've never previously noticed. Just one of these could open the door to lasting happiness. CAT therapists don't promise to cure you in sixteen weeks, but they'll give you the tools to finish the job.

You'll need to do some homework between sessions, usually monitoring thoughts, actions and feelings. These notes are used in CAT to give you better understanding of how to make positive changes. Your last three sessions look at ending therapy and how this might affect you, especially if other endings or good-byes have been difficult. As well as talking about endings, you'll consolidate key themes from your work together.

23. Restoration day

If you're suffering from chronic, long-term stress and burnout is imminent, here is your emergency plan.

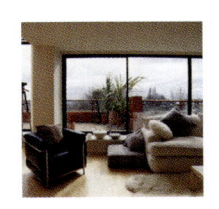

Book yourself a day out. By tomorrow, you will feel rested, stronger and more in control. Remember that if you don't look after yourself, you will have nothing left to give to others. The restoration day is based on three principles: 1) replenish your body by giving it rest; 2) rest your brain by focusing on your body; and 3) nourish your soul with healthy simple food that will replenish the nutrients stripped away by stress.

When you wake, acknowledge that this day will be different. Today you are going to shift the emphasis onto relaxation and releasing tension and replacing what stress has drained away from your body. When you get up, stretch for 10 minutes. A few yoga stretches are good, but it doesn't matter as long as you try to stretch every muscle in your body. It's not a work out, it's a reminder – you have a body: it carries tension and pain. Feel the cricks draining out.

Try a fruit smoothie for breakfast. Imagine the vitamin C zooming around your body replacing the

Defining idea...

'Rest as soon as there is pain.'
HIPPOCRATES

Here's an idea for you...

Go to bed at 9.30 p.m. today and every day this week if you can manage it. Don't watch TV if you're not tired – read or listen to music. People who do this have turned around their stress levels in a week.

levels depleted by stress. Eat lightly and avoid foods that strain digestion too much. Spend the rest of the morning outside in natural surroundings. Ideally, lie on the grass and stare at the sky. Let your mind drift off. Or walk in the countryside or a park. If you really can't bear to be still, do some gardening.

For lunch, have a huge salad combining every colour of vegetable you can think of: more vitamin C. This meal must include one absolute treat – a glass of wine, a dish of ice cream, a piece of chocolate. Afterwards, curl up on your sofa. Watch a favourite movie, or a comedy show. A weepie can be great because a good cry is very therapeutic.

You should be hungry but feeling light by dinner time. Eat another pile of vegetables, again following the 'eat a rainbow' advice given above. Present your food beautifully and eat it by candlelight so your evening starts in serene mood.

24. At the peak

High self-esteem makes you happier. Revving yours up should be easy if you follow these simple rules.

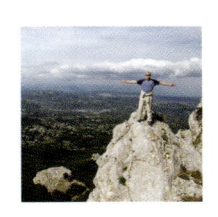

Self-esteem's a combination of how much you think you're worth and how accepted you feel. High self-esteem helps you cope with setbacks and makes you more immune to depression. Value yourself highly, and you'll also be more creative, resilient and successful.

You've probably noticed different bits of your life go well at different times. Work's going well, you're getting on well with your partner, but all your kitchen appliances break down, one after another. No rhyme or reason to it; just life. The trouble is, if your self-esteem is all tied up with one bit of your life, when that bit goes badly, you're more at risk of depression. So, spread your assets. Work on other areas, like friendships, hobbies and sports. That way, if you're made redundant and your wife leaves you for an older man, your prize marrows and pals from the allotment might just see you through.

Even high-flyers can see themselves negatively because they compare themselves with other people in their league. This makes them lose

Defining idea...

'The things we hate about ourselves aren't more real than things we like about ourselves.'
ELLEN GOODMAN, journalist

Here's an idea for you...

Forget perfection: try setting your goals below your usual threshold for a week and see your self-esteem soar. When we set our goals too high, we hardly ever reach them. When we do, it's amazing, but the rest of the time, we feel worthless.

sight of how well they're doing. They are tiddlers in a shoal of equally high achievers. Being a big fish in a small pond is a great way to bump up your self-esteem, so spend more time doing the things you know you do well.

Friends influence the way we see ourselves. A jealous girlfriend might persuade you your bum looks gigantic in those jeans, just because she can't afford them. Ditching friends who make you feel bad is an effective self-esteem booster. Time for an address book audit. Look through your chums and ask yourself two serious questions: Who helps me feel good about myself? Who makes me feel small and insignificant? Be ruthless: cut ties with those people in the latter category.

Another must is to snuff out that little voice inside that whispers things like 'You never do anything right'. Next time the voice pipes up, think back carefully over what happened, and remind yourself of all the details. That should shut it up.

25. The clinic is open

You know you're stressed and you know it's affecting your health. It's time to do something about it.

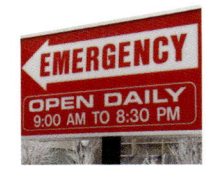

Stress hits your hormones hard. And this can make its effects felt in the darnedest places.

Bad digestion? Adrenaline slows digestion so food hangs around in your gut for longer, leading to constipation and bloating. Conversely, noradrenaline acts to open up the bowel, which leads to diarrhoea. That's one reason why irritable bowel syndrome (IBS), which is often stress-related, can manifest itself with apparently opposite symptoms. *Take action:* Probiotic supplements boost the good bacteria in the gut and this will help combat the effects of the stress hormones. Your doctor may be able to offer further help.

Spots or dry skin? When you're stressed, your body diverts resources away from areas that don't contribute to its immediate survival – like your skin. Stress also makes women produce more testosterone

Defining idea...

'On the plus side, death is one of the few things that can be done just as easily lying down.'
WOODY ALLEN

Here's an idea for you...

Make a list of your top seven people. Think of how important your continued good health is to them. if you can't do it for yourself, those we love can be powerful motivation.

and that can cause spots. *Take action:* A multivitamin will help fill the gap in your nutritional needs. Omega 3 and 6 fats help dry skin.

Always tired? The hormones that regulate sleep include serotonin and melatonin – and both are affected by periods of stress. Stress also causes high levels of the hormone cortisol, which keeps you alert. Not useful at bedtime. *Take action:* Your doctor may be able to help with a short-term prescription. Sleeping tablets if only taken for a very short period at a time of crisis are not addictive.

Weight gain? Yes, stress and weight gain are related. Stress is thought to interfere with the action of insulin, which regulates energy release. This could be contributing to a condition known as 'insulin resistance', which leads to weight gain along with an increased likelihood of other dangerous conditions such as diabetes. *Take action:* Dieting won't necessarily help with insulin resistance if you are still eating the wrong kind of carbohydrates – mainly processed ones. Get healthy carbs from vegetables and eat them with a little protein or fat. This slows down their breakdown and, thus, insulin release into your bloodstream.

Ultimately, getting on top of the causes of your stress will help with all these problems.

Idea 26 – **Know what to do**

26. Know what to do

Are you in need of ways to cope with problems that trigger depression? Try these tried and trusted strategies.

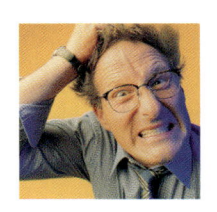

Problems with partners, friends, health, work or money often trigger depression. So, it's hardly surprising that problem-solving skills reduce anxiety and hopelessness. Try this formula.

Start by writing down problems that are contributing to your depression. Melika did this and her list was as follows: Having lots of arguments with dad; Struggling to keep up credit repayments; Feel lonely and cut off from friends; Being bullied by my boss.

Overwhelmed with problems? Pick one at a time. Nobody can solve all their problems in one hit. So choose the problem that troubles you most immediately. Melika starred her last item.

Identify different options by brainstorming. Yes, it sounds like a gimmick for advertising moguls, but it works. Get out the flipchart – or at least a big bit of paper – and scribble down as many possible solutions as you can.

Defining idea...

'A problem well-stated is a problem half-solved.'
CHARLES FRANKLIN KETTERING, American inventor

Here's an idea for you...

Instead of ruminating endlessly on your problems, pick one or two critical issues and ask a friend to help you brainstorm solutions. Bouncing ideas off each other will help you come up with a richer list.

These questions should help: What have you heard that's worked before? If my best friend had this problem, what would I suggest? Include anything – even zany or outlandish stuff can help you think quickly and creatively. Melika was depressed after months of bullying by her boss. Here are her more serious brainstorm options: Stab boss with letter opener; Stay out of his way; Confront him; Tell his boss.

Examine every solution, weighing up pros and cons. When you've got a list of options, think through the pros and cons of each. Melika didn't fancy spending time in prison so she focused on the last two.

Pick the solution that has more pros than the others. As you think of the pros and cons, run each option through this two-question filter: Will it help? Can I do it?

Plan steps you'll take to put your chosen solution into action and go for it. So what happened with Melika? She confronted her boss. He denied everything and became more aggressive. So, she went for her second option, speaking to his superior. It turns out he'd bullied before. He was given his marching orders. She's much happier.

Idea 26 – **Know what to do**

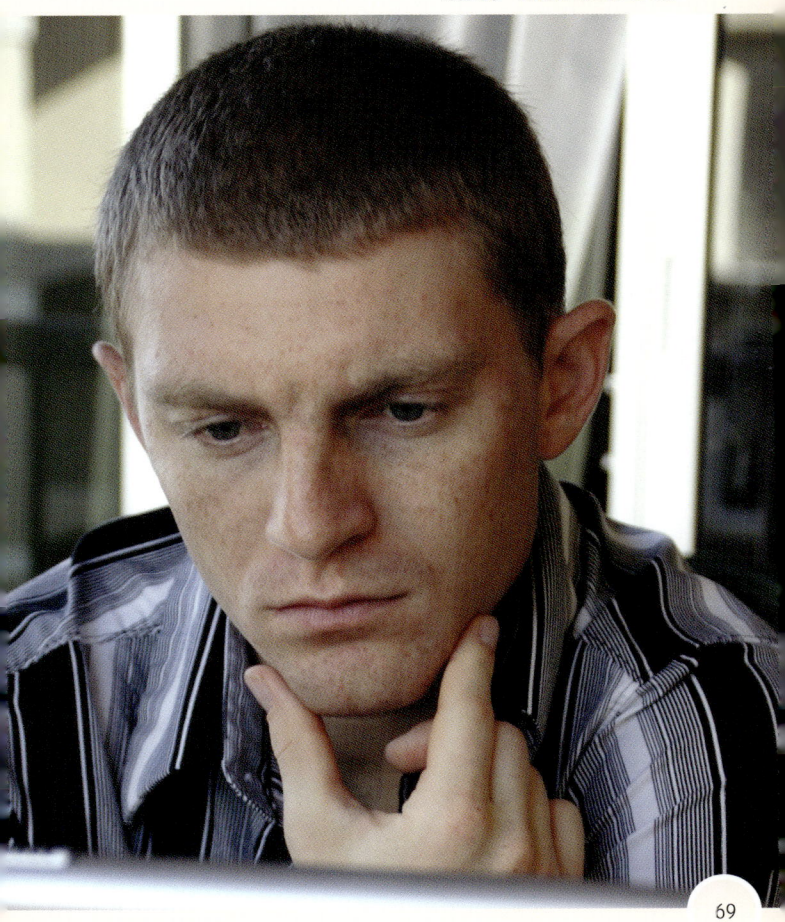

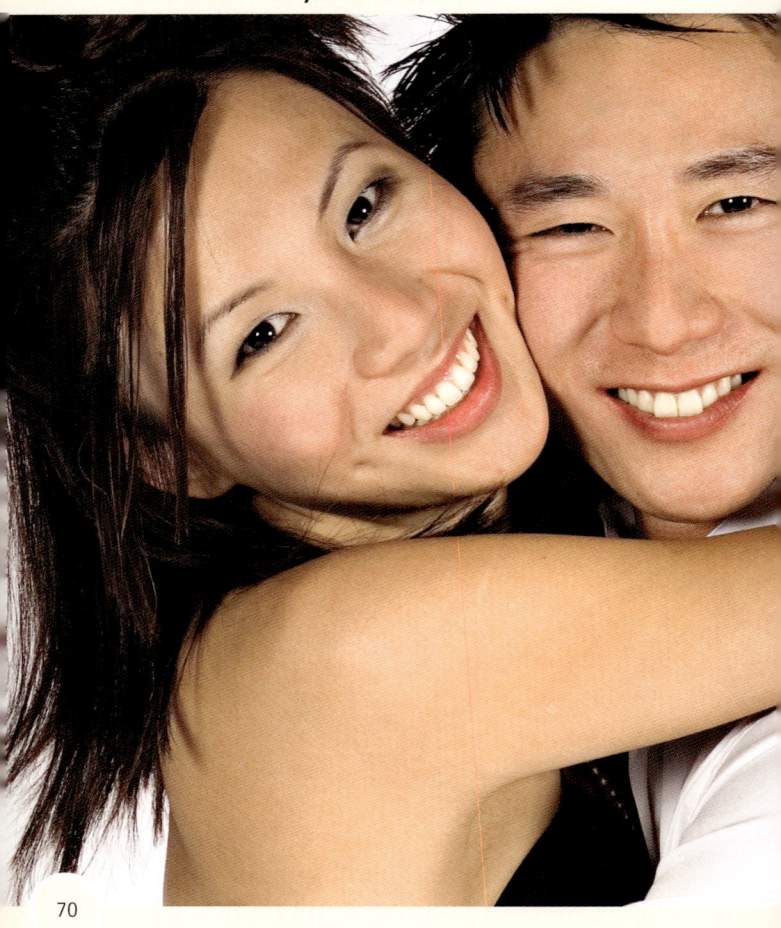

27. How to be loved

The need for approval can be a source of personal stress. Get a warm glow from dishing it out rather than seeking it.

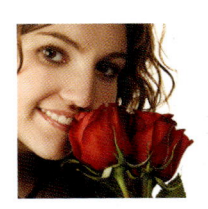

We are approval-seeking missiles. We start off wanting a smile from mum for playing nicely or using the potty. And it's a direct line from that to remodelling your house so it's bigger than the neighbours' and stealing your mate's ideas at work to impress the boss. This constant need for approval is a major source of stress.

People often satisfy this need through feeling superior by lording it over other people they consider inferior to themselves. This is the origin of most success-driven behaviours. And it's why many of us spend much of the time feeling like schmucks. When we're comparing ourselves with other people – what they have, what they do – we feel less than equal. That sets up a deep anxiety that usually leads to you trying even harder to make other people acknowledge your worth.

And one day you wake up and no one seems to like you much – not even your kids (who've probably

Defining idea...

'We can secure other people's approval, if we do right and try hard; but our own is worth a hundred of it, and no way has been found out of securing that.'
MARK TWAIN

Here's an idea for you...

When you're in a situation where you feel intimidated, pretend the other person is a guest in your home and your job is to make them feel comfortable. The host/hostess scenario creates an equal relationship and you forget to feel self-conscious.

suffered your surreptitious 'superiority' routine more than most). In fact, the success-driven behaviours that we use to win approval are likely to result in the direct opposite. How do we break free?

If somebody's trying to make you feel worthless, try to work out what's motivating their behaviour. This is not the same as worrying about what they think about you. Try to see into their hearts – can you see any stresses that could be making them act mean? Then do your best to make them feel better. Remember that all of us are approval-seeking missiles – including the people acting out their inferiority/superiority thing on you.

If you stop feeling the need to act superior, you'll stop feeling inferior You will speak to people straightforwardly, refusing to be intimidated by 'superiors' and declining to play the damaging game of putting yourself in some pecking order. You will be a person walking confidently through life spreading grace and goodwill. You will love the world and it will love you right back.

28. Don't panic

Depression and anxiety go hand in glove. Fight back by managing panic attacks and all those irrational fears.

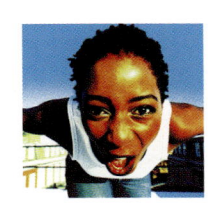

Depression's hard to cope with and it means the small stuff is more likely to wind you up. Anxiety is caused when your primeval fight-or-flight mechanism gets activated. It kicks in when you feel under threat. Low-level stress is essential for survival, enabling you to produce work to high standards, but adding extra stress when you've already reached your peak can have catastrophic results. Typically, tiredness is the first sign. Exhaustion and illness follow if stress continues unchecked.

Racing or pounding heartbeat, chest pain, dizziness, tingling hands, a feeling that something unimaginably horrifying is about to happen, fear of going mad, fear of dying? If you've had some of these symptoms, it was a panic attack. They last about ten minutes, and they're one of the most frightening and upsetting things you can go through. What can you do about them?

Defining idea...

'Anxiety is a thin stream of fear trickling through the mind. If encouraged, it cuts a channel into which all other thoughts are drained.'
ARTHUR SOMERS ROCHE, writer

Here's an idea for you...

Visit a self-help or support group to discover how other people have overcome anxiety. You may well find they have developed techniques that work well for you too.

The first thing to remember is that these symptoms are harmless: they can't make you have a heart attack or stroke, and you're not going crazy. They happen because your body has had a false alarm, kicking you into fight-or-flight mode. Breathing deeply and slowly counteracts the effects of this reaction. Many people fear they'll faint, making a fool of themselves, but fear not. When the fight-or-flight response kicks in, your blood pressure rises, making fainting physiologically impossible.

Phobias – irrational fears – make matters worse. Sufferers know that things like the dark, dogs or lifts can't harm them, but they still feel irrationally scared. Cognitive behaviour therapy (CBT) can help you cope with anxiety-provoking situations, often by exposing you to them. This might seem counterintuitive but it helps tackle the symptoms. CBT shows you that many terrifying thoughts are harmless. As you learn to no longer fear the sensations and scary thoughts, you become less and less afraid of panic.

29. Watch out: iceberg!

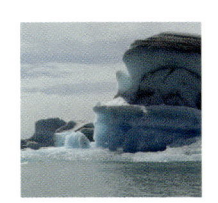

Like the *Titanic*, you can be sailing true, then crunch! You're sunk. That's the effect of iceberg stress.

As many as one-third of people admit they have been laid low out of nowhere with some mysterious stress-related illness. There are always signs, but we rarely pay attention to them until they are dangerous. It's possible to go on for a long time with low-grade stress symptoms before they clobber you.

The signs will be there, but are you paying attention? A recent study discovered that 48% of people admitted to being irritable because they were stressed, 44% didn't sleep, 35% were permanently exhausted. But then there was the 19% who claimed that stress had no effect on their health at all – they're the true workaholics.

Below are a few questions worth asking yourself. It will give you an idea of where you fall in the stress gradient, stage 1 being less difficult

Defining idea...

'People who don't know how to keep themselves healthy ought to have the decency to get themselves buried, and not waste time about it.'
HENRIK IBSEN

Here's an idea for you...

Write down your ten emotional highs in the last month and ten emotional lows. If it's easy to think of the bad times, but not the good ones, you may be more stressed than you realised. Feeling emotionally defunct is a sign that burnout could be closer than you think.

than stage 3. Those with stage 1 may be showing mild signs of iceberg stress, those with stage 2 moderate symptoms. Exercise, sleep, a decent diet and – most of all – changing your habits will do a lot to help. Those on stage 3 should consult their doctor and consider overhauling their lifestyle, pronto. They almost certainly have iceberg stress. Test yourself today.

Stage 1 – snowball: Do you often get minor skin blemishes such as cold sores? Do you get cravings for sweet, sugary foods? Do you experience energy slumps?

Stage 2 – snowman: Are you prone to spots that don't appear to be related to puberty or the menopause? Do you get every bug going and find it hard to recover from illness? Do you get constipation or suffer tummy problems, such as bloating or acid reflux? Are you inexplicably overweight? Have you lost weight because you're just too busy?

Stage 3 – the whole damn iceberg: Do you suffer from exhaustion all the time? Do you suffer from eczema that is getting worse? Do you have irritable bowel syndrome that's not under control? Do you suffer from high blood pressure, palpitations or dizziness?

30. Natural highs

Poised to pop a herbal helper? The idea of nature's Prozac may be hard to swallow but it might just save your life.

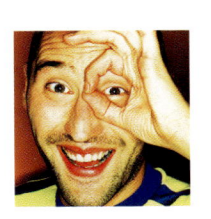

Lavender, borage and ginkgo biloba have been plugged as herbal cures for depression. Some so-called natural remedies do deliver what they promise on the label but others are ineffective impostors or even a toxic rip-off. Good scientific evidence that herbal treatment works is pretty scant so it was a welcome surprise when a little yellow shrub named after a saint caused a stir in the *British Medical Journal*. Researchers showed it to be effective in treating people with mild or moderate depression.

What was the magic weed? *Hypericum perforatum*, known by most of us as St John's Wort. It grows in many parts of the world and it has been used as a herbal remedy for around two thousand years. The active ingredient, hypericin, works on brain chemistry like conventional antidepressants. It corrects the imbalance in serotonin that occurs when you're depressed.

Rigorous scientific trials mean there's a lot to be said for conventional

Defining idea...

'The cheering effects of herbs and alliums cannot be too often reiterated.'
PATIENCE GRAY, cookery author

Here's an idea for you...

Talk through the pros and cons of taking St John's Wort with your doctor. If you decide to go for it, you'll need to take it for at least four weeks before it starts to lift your mood.

medicine. But, if you've ever taken them, you'll know conventional antidepressants cause a lot of side effects. The good news is that St John's Wort has fewer side effects than non-herbal antidepressants. However, some people find their skin burns more easily in the sun. If you're taking St John's Wort, you might feel sick, tired or form a deep and meaningful relationship with your lavatory. St John's Wort also plays dirty tricks in your liver. It interacts with cytochrome P450, which means half a pharmacist's stock – including the contraceptive pill – won't work properly if you take them with St John's Wort.

In the UK, it isn't licensed and so can't be prescribed, but you might be able to buy St John's Wort without a prescription in health food shops or pharmacies. However, depression is a serious illness and it's never a good idea to self-medicate. Check with your doctor to find out whether St John's Wort will be a life saver for you.

31. Stress is others

Other people can sometimes leach the self-esteem out of you. Learn how to deal with these black holes.

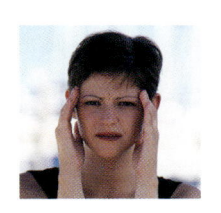

All around you are the energy black holes – people who are unhappy, negative or angry and who would like nothing more than to drag you into their stressful world. Other people have their own agenda. You can't know what it is and you can't change it. The only thing you can change is your attitude towards them when you interact.

If your life is littered with difficult people who seem out to get you, then it might suggest there's something wrong with your expectations. However, most times, it's not your problem – it's theirs.

There is a surprisingly telling little exercise that you can do in five minutes on the back of a napkin. It may give you shock. Make a list of the people with whom you have regular contact. Then divide that list into three categories:

The energizers: They look after you in every way. They give great advice. They bring happiness to your life.

Defining idea...

'A healthy male adult bore consumes each year one and a half times his own weight in other people's patience.'

JOHN UPDIKE

Here's an idea for you...

When you feel surrounded by bullies at work, ask yourself some important questions. Do you work hard, pitch up, do your best? Are you fair and impartial, and pleasant as you can be? Yes? Then you're doing all you can so don't waste time worrying about what they're saying about you.

The neutral: They're OK – neither great nor bad.

The drainers: They're users – people who don't deliver, let you down and bring you down. They also include gossips, people whose conversation is sexist or racist and bitchy, sarcastic types whose conversation, no matter how entertaining, makes you feel bad about yourself afterwards.

You know what we're going to say. Maximise time with the energisers. Look for them when you enter a room and gravitate towards them whether you've been introduced or not. We all know these people when we meet them. If you have too many neutrals, think how you can bring more energisers into your life.

And the drainers? Your time with them should be strictly limited. And if some of them are your closest friends, your family, your lover, you need to think about that very closely. You may feel unable to cut them out now (although that is an option) but you can limit the time they are allowed to suck you into their world.

32. Just say no

Are you a people pleaser, swamped by always saying 'yes'? Perfect the art of polite refusal and show depression the door.

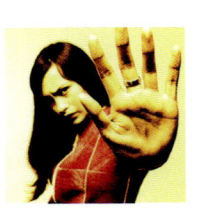

Fed up with being taken for granted? It's hard to say no when you feel pitiful or worthless. Maybe you feel you've no control over what happens. The snag is, helplessness feeds depression. Imagine responding to a friend's cries for sympathy like this:

"If you're a people pleaser, you'll know that if you always say 'yes' to others, you're soon taken for granted. Learning to say 'no' puts you back in control and stops the feelings of powerlessness that feed depression. Remember that saying 'no' doesn't mean you're snubbing people, just that you're declining demands."

When you say 'no', think of it as a polite refusal. Keep it short and stick to your point. Here are some nice ways of saying 'no': *Let's go for a swim.* Sorry, I really don't enjoy swimming. *Fancy coming back for a coffee?* No, I can't stay out late as I've got an early

Defining idea...

'The art of leadership is saying no, not saying yes. It is very easy to say yes.'

TONY BLAIR

Here's an idea for you...

If you've been talked out of previous refusals, try starting sentences with the word no. It's harder to backtrack if it's the first word you say.

start tomorrow. Try using body language to back up what you say. Shaking your head, while saying 'no', is a good start.

Still squirming at the thought of saying 'no'? Take a leaf out of Jessie's book. Jessie's a champion cake baker, a teacher and single mum of three. She was often asked to bake cakes for charity sales, birthdays and weddings. In the past, she always said 'yes', often staying up ridiculously late to get the baking or decorating finished. A hobby that had been the source of so much pleasure started to stress her out. Now when she's asked to bake, she sighs, and says, 'You know, I'd really love to, but, I've just got too much on. Maybe next time.' If you're uneasy about an outright no, how about presenting a trade-off like, 'I might just be able to do that, if you babysat for me/cleaned my car/did my shopping.'

Avoid changing your mind, however much demanding, imploring or flattery you face. In time you'll become skilled at not only saying 'no', but also saying 'no' without feeling guilty.

33. Conquer obstacles

For every action, there's a payback. Work out the payback to drain away a lot of stress from a situation.

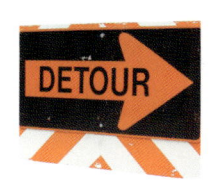

OK, this is a brutal one. You're being asked for sympathy but cruel thoughts are in your mind. It's called the truth. Imagine responding to a friend's cries for sympathy like this:

"You're using work as an excuse to avoid going home, and it's pretty obvious to everyone what's going on, including the folks back home. Maybe that's why the family are so unpleasant when you bother to show up? You're single, over 40, and unhappy about it? You made the choices even if they didn't feel like choices at the time. It was your choice to run from the people who wanted to commit to you in favour of those people who didn't want to commit to you – all of whom, incidentally, you invited into your life."

Of course, we rarely ever say these things. However, if we were really serious about sorting out our stress levels, we all could start by taking our share of the responsibility for creating them.

Defining idea...

'I think of a hero as someone who understands the degree of responsibility that comes with his freedom.'
BOB DYLAN

Here's an idea for you...

Make a game out of working out the payback for your actions on a daily basis. You'll find it interesting to observe when you're 'running a racket' (i.e. kidding yourself).

When you realise the great truth that you create a lot of your stress by your choices, then you're in a position to work out what you're getting from the situation. Sometimes the payback is worth the stress. You choose to look after your ill child. That's stressful but the payback is, of course, self-evident. Others are trickier and take great honesty. Sacked from your job? But, remember: even when the job began to look iffy, you decided not to leave because the pay was good and it was near your home.

So whatever your stress source, look carefully at what choices of yours led to it. It is incredibly liberating to recognise that in every single thing you do, every single relationship you have, every single habit you have, you are getting some sort of payback *or you wouldn't do it*. Acknowledging the payback gives us immense self-awareness. Obstacles melt away because we stop blaming everyone else. Once we're self-aware we tend to change of our own free will. The truth will set you free.

34. Reboot

What you think about what's happening affects the way you feel. A positive spin will improve your mood.

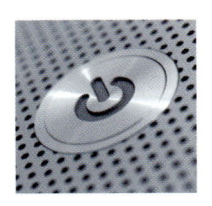

When you're depressed, you're more inclined to see the worst in yourself, the world and your future. This negative spin takes several guises:

- *Assuming the worst.* My wife hasn't phoned. She must have been killed in a car crash on the way home from work.

- *Assuming everything is going badly when only one thing has gone badly.* I failed that exam so there's no point going to college tomorrow. I'll never get a decent job.

- *Focusing on the bad stuff, while ignoring the good stuff.* That novel I had published is bound to be remaindered because there's a typo on page fifteen.

- *Putting a negative slant on everything positive.* My boss only gave me a good appraisal because he feels sorry for me.

Defining idea...

'If you never change your mind, why have one?'

EDWARD DE BONO

Here's an idea for you...

Try this exercise. Jot down the last thing that left you feeling miserable. Draw a line down the page. On the left-hand side, list any negative spin you might have put on it. On the right, come up with a level-headed thought to replace it.

If you're thinking like this, it's time to reboot your hard drive. This requires swapping the negative spin for more balanced thinking and it takes some practice. The trick is to balance every negative notion with a more level-headed one.

As an example, take two friends, Melanie and Jilly, whose different thought processes lead to chalk-and-cheese reactions to the same experience. One Saturday, Melanie went to her first singles party with Elaine. Elaine met a tall, dark guy and was asked on a date. Melanie didn't. Melanie thought: Elaine is prettier than me. I'll never get asked out. Nobody understands me. I am worthless. She became depressed, which lasted for two weeks. Jilly also went to her first singles party with Elaine. Elaine met a tall, fair guy and was asked on a date. Jilly didn't. Jilly thought: Elaine's been here before, she knows how to get a date. It'll be my turn next time. Anyway, I had fun dancing, even though I didn't meet anybody. She was mildly disappointed, but got over it by Sunday afternoon.

Jilly's more realistic thinking is obviously going to produce a better mood. If you can rephrase thoughts, making them seem more optimistic, you'll make major inroads on your depression.

35. Life-work balance

It should be life-work balance, not work-life. And that's what achieving it entails – a life-work.

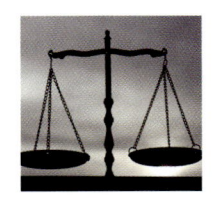

One of the most pernicious things about stress is the way we don't notice how it switches our attention away from what we value and love in life until it's too late. So here are some pointers to test if stress is stomping all over your life-work balance…

Do you feel like your day is spent dealing with difficult people and difficult tasks? Do you feel that those you love don't have a clue what's going on with you? Do you regularly make time for activities that nourish your soul? Do you feel you could walk out of your house and no one would notice you were gone until the mortgage had to be paid?

You guessed it – number 3 was the trick question! Answer 'yes' to that one and you're probably okay. Answer 'yes' to the rest and you could be in trouble. In a nutshell: make sure you're putting time and effort into the people and activities

Defining idea…

'The best and safest thing is to keep a balance in your life, acknowledge the great powers around us and in us. If you can do that, and live that way, you are really a wise man.'
EURIPIDES

Here's an idea for you...

Designate Saturday 'family' day and Sunday afternoon 'selfish' time. We can usually find an hour or so on Sunday afternoon to spend on ourselves – just don't let it get filled with chores or your partner's agenda.

that make your heart sing and it really is very difficult to buckle under the effect of stress.

Everyone assumes that all we need is less work and more life, then all would be in harmonious balance. Not so. Where it has gone all wrong for so many – women especially – is that they've cleared enough time for the 'life' part of the equation but not taken into account that home-making isn't necessarily restful or enjoyable. Your children may be the reason you get out of bed in the morning but you need to accept that spending more time with them is not necessarily any less stressful than work. More time with yourself probably is.

It's true – if you don't look after yourself, you can't look after anyone else. A few minutes of selfishness every day is enough to make a profound difference in your ability to achieve a life balance that works. Try it.

36. Rant and rave

It's not getting angry that's the problem, it's how you express it. Gain advantage by transforming rage into passion.

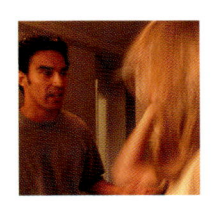

Depression stops you doing things. It drains away motivation, drive and energy. Anger, on the other hand, induces and even compels us to action. Some believe that it's good to make depressed people angry for this exact reason. Sigmund Freud went one further, saying depression is anger turned inwards against yourself.

Many people are scared that an angry outburst will ruin a relationship irretrievably. Acting in the heat of the moment means you are more likely to be impulsive or rash. Nobody wants to be a bully, so learning to calm down and channel your anger helps you use it in a positive way.

If you're angry with the snotty kids who keep vandalising the bus stop outside your house, getting angry can be helpful. Instead of charging out there and getting a criminal record for assaulting them, use your

Defining idea...

'Heat not a furnace for your foe so hot that it do singe yourself.'
WILLIAM SHAKESPEARE, *King Henry VIII*

Here's an idea for you...

Each time you get angry, spend some time afterwards seeing if you can identify any common triggers. Discovering what or who presses your buttons means you can deal with anger in a more constructive, less destructive way.

rage constructively. Get a neighbourhood watch scheme going or organise a petition for CCTV at the bus stop.

Next time you feel your blood about to boil over, try these techniques. First, walk away to give yourself some essential cooling-off time. It also distracts you temporarily, which can help give you a sense of perspective. It takes most people twenty minutes to calm down, so be prepared to count to ten a few times.

Or you could pretend you're sitting opposite the person who's made your blood boil. Let rip and tell them what's on your mind. Now sit in their chair and imagine what your rant sounded like. Can you see it from their perspective? If you can do this, you're more likely to respond in an assertive rather than aggressive way. What's the difference? Being assertive means standing up for yourself rather than attacking or hurting others.

Try writing a letter to the person you're angry with. Dump your inhibitions and say exactly how you feel. Be as abusive as you like. But then tear the letter up. Wait for a couple of days and then write a more measured letter that you can post. Are you feeling calmer? Brilliant.

37. Speed parenting

Children pick up adult stress like a dry sponge soaks up water. That's when you need focused parental skills.

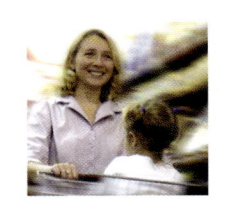

Calm parents usually means calm kids. When you're frazzled, they reflect it and have a horrible tendency to get bad tempered, argumentative, clingy and sick. That's because stress is contagious. Most parents know the rule of 'reverse serendipity' that guarantees it's on the days when your car gets broken into and your job depends on you delivering a fabulous (and as yet unprepared) presentation that your kids will play up to the max.

Up to the age of about ten, children think their parents' stress is their fault. After that, they're less egocentric and recognise that outside factors cause it. However, they can still feel it's their responsibility to sort out the problem for mum or dad. But since your twelve-year-olds can't possibly stop your boss firing you or your computer crashing, their efforts to lighten your load will only be a partial success. Children discover that their efforts aren't making you happy and that can transfer into adult feelings of guilt and low self-esteem.

Defining idea...

'There is no way to be a perfect parent, but thousands of ways of being a great one.'
ANON

Here's an idea for you...

Next time you talk to a child get on their level, eye to eye. They respond better. Kneel when they're toddlers; stand on a stool when they're teenagers.

A short-term answer is to explain that you're stressed out. Tell them why, but also show them that you're working out a way to handle it. Your competence in the face of a stressful day is an invaluable lesson for later life. Spelling it all out goes a long way to reassuring them.

And on those days when it's all going pear-shaped, your kids are being unbearable and not letting you get on with what you have to do, then the best advice is to give them what they want – your time. Pleading for an hour of peace won't work, but ten minutes of concentrating on them – a quick game, a chat, a cuddle and a story – calms them down and they tend to wander off and leave you alone.

In the longer term, besides demonstrating your competence in handling stress, the other side of stress-proofing your kids is to make them feel secure. The more secure your children are, the better they'll be able to handle stress for the rest of their lives – even the stress that's caused by you.

38. When drugs fail

For a third of people, antidepressants don't work. If you're one of them, don't despair.

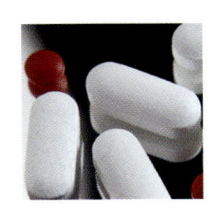

Ask yourself: 'Am I really depressed?' No doubt you feel unhappy, tired and don't enjoy the things you used to love doing, but there may be another explanation for your dejection. If the drugs aren't dealing with your depression, it may be time to revisit your original diagnosis.

An underactive thyroid gland could be the problem. Low thyroid hormone levels can cause dreadful depression so it's important to get yours checked and treated if need be. Vigorously correcting even borderline thyroid hormone levels has an immense effect on low mood.

Sienna's depression didn't get any better with treatment. She felt tearful and drained, but also had a bit of a sore throat she couldn't shake off. Her eyes looked puffy, but she thought it was because she had cried so much. Then her doctor did a blood test that showed she had glandular fever. As this got

Defining idea...

'Reality is a crutch for people who can't cope with drugs.'
LILY TOMLIN, actor

Here's an idea for you...

Assuming you've been to the doctor and there's nothing else going on, hand on heart, do you always take your medication? People often forgot. Look for things you could do to remind yourself, like crossing off a day on the calendar or putting a tick in your diary. Could you set up a daily reminder on your mobile phone?

better, she stopped feeling so debilitated and dejected.

Ernie was feeling depressed and the tablets and counselling didn't do much good. He lost his appetite and his clothes hung off him. After several weeks he turned yellow and his skin itched horribly. Ernie actually had pancreatic cancer. Don't panic, though: most people with depression don't have cancer. However, around 10–20% of depression is set off by another illness, so it's important to rule out bodily causes for your low mood.

It's worth checking out with your prescriber whether you are on a high enough dose or if you've you been on this dose for long enough to expect a noticeable effect. If it's a yes to both, it's probably time for a different drug. You could also try something called augmentation. This means adding in another drug to make your antidepressant work better. There are a number of different drugs used for this, and it needs to be properly tailored to your requirements by a professional. If you're not yet having a regular 'talking' treatment, or seeking a second opinion, there's never been a better time to get that going.

39. Work to rules

Take control. Don't let your working day be hijacked by others. The secret is to have your goals clearly in mind.

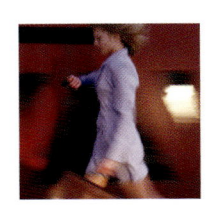

Don't be slave to a daily 'to-do' list. Look at the bigger picture. On Monday morning, think: 'What are my goals for this week?' Break each goal into smaller tasks. This helps you prioritise so that the tricky things, or tasks that depend on other people's input, don't sink to the back of your consciousness. It also means you are alert to all that you have to do and you're not overwhelmed by one task at the beginning of the week.

If your job demands creativity, cordon off your most creative periods so that you can concentrate on your projects. Don't let them be impinged upon by meetings and phone calls that could be done anytime. Make the phone call you're dreading – right now. Have meetings in the morning when people are frisky and want to whizz through stuff so they can get on with their day.

Defining idea...

'Take a note of the balls you're juggling. As you keep your work, health, family, friends and spirit in the air, remember that work is a rubber ball and will bounce back if you drop it. All the rest are made of glass; drop one of them and it will be irrevocably scuffed, tarnished or even smashed.'
JON BRIGGS, voice-over supremo

Here's an idea for you...

Create a 'virtual you' if you're getting stressed out in the office by the demands of others. When you're an administrative lynchpin, set up a shared file where people can go to find the information or resources they'd usually get from you.

Talk to other people on the phone when it suits you, not them. Limit your calls to three times a day. Make your calls first thing when people are gagging for a coffee. If someone isn't there, leave a message and ask them to call you back in your next 'phone period'. Just before lunch is good. With grumbling stomachs, neither of you will linger over the call. Your other 'phone time' should be around 4.30 p.m. for similar reasons. (Use the same strategy with emails.)

Of course, you can't limit phone calls completely to these times but most of us have some control over incoming calls. You could politely say 'Sorry, I'm in the middle of something', and tell the caller when you'll be free. Most people offer to call back, saving you the hassle of calling them. No one minds that if their call isn't urgent.

Idea 39 – **Work to rules**

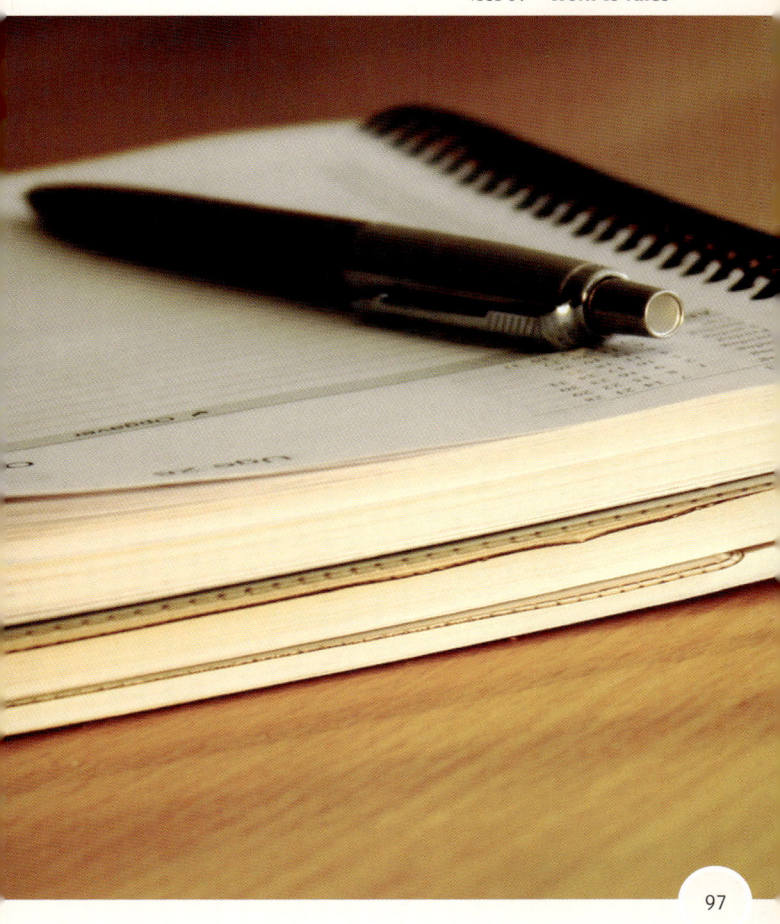

52 Brilliant Ideas – **Heal your troubled mind**

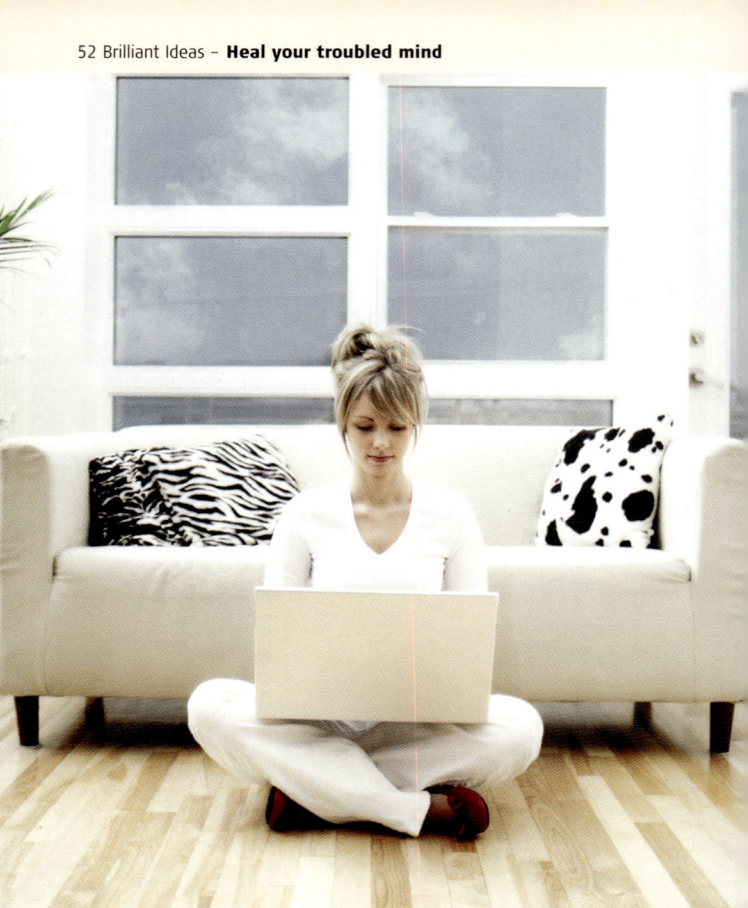

40. Toil and trouble

Work is often blamed for stressing us out. However, there's a flip side. Hard graft does have healing powers.

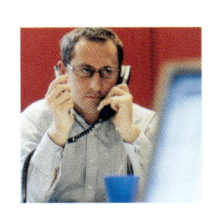

True, our jobs can make us deeply unhappy, but we mustn't forget that having nothing to do swiftly drives people into a state of nihilism – staring into oblivion, hoping to become extinct. Consider these reasons why work works as a depression buster: it can raise our self-esteem and make us feel appreciated; it gives us a sense of purpose and a structure for our days (and lives); mastering a series of goals makes us feel good; it offers a source of distraction from depressing thoughts; it's often a good place to make friends and hang out with them; and working can, sometimes, be fun. Let's admit it: the money you earn helps too. Cash gives you control over your life and means you can make the sort of decisions you can't make if you're on welfare, like 'Sun or skiing?' Anybody's who's been on the dole for a while knows all too well that without wages, it's hard to plan ahead. You're dropped by society and robbed of your identity.

Defining idea...

'Happiness does not come from doing easy work but from the afterglow of satisfaction that comes after the achievement of a difficult task that demanded our best.'

THEODORE I. RUBIN, psychiatrist and author

Here's an idea for you...

Imagine you're interviewing prospective candidates for your dream job. What are you looking for in the perfect candidate? Now imagine you're applying. Revamp your CV accordingly. Tackle the interview questions. Would you give yourself the job? If not, what more do you need? What courses can you take? Who can help you?

So, you've been off work with stress or depression for a long time but now you're ready to return – but anxious. How can you smooth your resurrection? If your employers are supportive, why not discuss a graded return with your boss? It makes sense to go back, say, three days per week initially, building up to full time over a couple of months. Many employers are happy to do this. There are other ways to take some of the pressure off. For instance, coming out of depression might mean you'll find it hard to concentrate on written work, while doing mechanical things like filing feels good. Get stuck into those tasks.

Avoid hiding at your desk during breaks – chat to colleagues so you'll feel more re-engaged. Enjoy the socialisation, and your paycheque: you've earned both.

41. Draw it out

Lost for words? The answer could be to explore your thoughts and emotions using sketches, paints, clay etc.

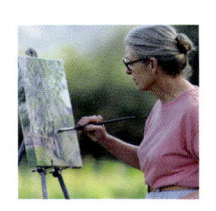

As well as being fun, art is a brilliant medium for healing heartache. Drawing, sketching, painting, sculpting, model making or collaging can release difficult feelings and help you cope with depression.

Art seems to serve a primal urge in many people – it's a powerful way of expressing yourself. Your pictures and models can be metaphors for distress and suffering. You don't even have to end up with a product – self-expression or 'making a mess' is valid in its own right. Art is about action, so it's great if you're feeling out of control. And, if you choose to share your work, it can also provide an insight into how you feel for family and friends.

The onus of art therapy is on healing rather than award-winning pictures or objects. For instance, researchers found that art therapy significantly reduced symptoms of depression in people with Alzheimer's disease. Art

Defining idea...

'Art is the stored honey of the human soul, gathered on wings of misery and travail.'
THEODORE DREISER, author

Here's an idea for you...

Squishing clay or rolling it flat is a great way of releasing pent-up anger. You can also use clay to model and squash a person or thing you wish you could be rid of.

gave them a way of expressing things that were beyond words or even comprehension.

Apart from being an enjoyable and gratifying activity, art opens your eyes. When you're depressed, you often stop noticing beauty. Sketching the roses makes you aware of pretty things again. Drawing heightens your awareness of sunsets, cityscapes and all sorts of natural and man-made objects, deepening your curiosity and injecting some colour into grey days.

People with depression are often perfectionists. Making collages with images and words cut or torn from magazines and newspapers is great if your inability to draw gets you down. When you're very depressed, painting or sketching can feel like too much effort, so collages are just the thing for tackling difficult themes.

One of the best things about this idea is that you often end up with something tangible. Many people find new meanings in their work when returning to art produced during depression. They recognise important undertones and nuances. Art therapists say this echoes changes in your recovery, showing you problems can be resolved.

42. All hands on deck

Having a regular massage can improve your quality of life and help you live with debilitating problems.

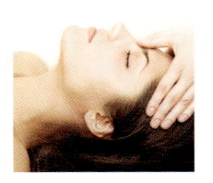

The sort of massage we're talking about here is soothing, simple and sensuous, and preferably performed by a trained massage therapist. It's a way of caressing, pressing and kneading your body to relieve tension and reduce pain. It leaves you feeling calm and cared for.

Being touched sensitively by another human being makes us feel warm and fuzzy. If we're deprived of touch, we often feel lonely and uneasy. Massage produces chemical changes in the brain and lowers levels of stress hormones. Teenage mums who received massage therapy, compared with those having relaxation therapy, were less depressed and less anxious, both by their own accounts and based on professional observations. Another study found that therapeutic massage eased depression among women who had lost a child.

Consider the reported benefits offered by massage. It reduces stress and tension; relieves pain; increases levels of serotonin (protecting against

Defining idea...

'In the absence of touching and being touched, people of all ages can sicken and grow touch starved.'
DIANE ACKERMAN, A Natural History of the Senses

Here's an idea for you...

Give acupuncture a try – some forms of depression seem to respond well to this treatment. Perhaps your doctor can recommend a local needle wizard.

depression) and endorphins (the body's natural pain killer); and strengthens the immune system. That's a potent list in anybody's book.

So, you want to go for a massage but you're confused by all the different names? Well, aromatherapy massage uses oils applied in long, flowing strokes, called 'effleurage'. These oils can be soothing or invigorating. Swedish massage is much more energetic. It's intended to energise by stimulating your circulation. Feldenkrais, Rolfing and Hellerwork are varieties of deep-tissue massage, which are great for easing strain out of the muscles and can help with injuries.

If you suffer tension headaches, massage your own forehead and feel stress melting away. Put the fingertips of your right hand on your right eyebrow. Pressing quite hard, slide your fingertips along each eyebrow until you reach your temple. Massage your temple by making small circles with your fingertips. Do the same with your left hand on your left eyebrow. You'll soon feel the benefit.

43. Sexual healing

Many depressed people lose interest in sex. Discover how to perk up your passions and your mood.

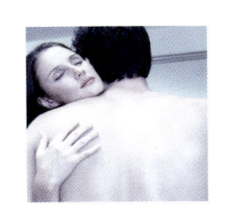

If you're looking for some really personal therapy, good sex is a lovely remedy. When you make love, your body releases natural feel-good chemicals called endorphins. They give you a euphoric buzz, lift your mood, increase pleasure and reduce pain. When you orgasm, your body releases a hormone called oxytocin, which makes you feel loved-up and blissful. All very well, but what if you're just not in the mood? Well, you're not alone – one-fifth of people have low or lost libidos.

Certain antidepressants can cause your sex drive to plummet to new depths. Selective serotonin reuptake inhibitors (SSRIs) are the commonest culprits. One of their side effects is that they zap one of our major sexual-pleasure chemicals, called dopamine. Ditching drugs is rarely your best strategy, but there are things you can do to reclaim your lust.

If your sex drive has driven off, rebuild the intimacy in your

Defining idea...

Arlene: You're crazy!
Phil: That's right! Not having sex for twelve years will do that to a person!
CITY SLICKERS

Here's an idea for you...

Remember the good feelings you had after making love? Rekindle those vibes. Swap your polyester bed sheets for silk or satin ones. Recreate your old memories – or try out some new fantasies.

relationship by kissing and cuddling. When did you last have a really good tongue tussle? Set aside time for regular passionate snuggles. Hug, kiss, enjoy forgotten sensations. Beforehand, you could serve up some oysters. Apart from their obvious similarities with women's bits, they're rich in zinc, a trace element essential for healthy sex organs. Caviar and mussels do the trick too.

Some sexperts suggest booking lovemaking times into your diaries, just as you'd schedule meetings. It might sound unromantic, but it can get you back into it. Avoid putting off sex because you haven't got time for a three-hour love-in. A quickie is better than nothing and the more sex you have, the more you'll feel like having.

Rev up your yearnings by making romance a top priority. Spoil yourself with sensual pleasures like silk pyjamas or a fur throw for your bed. Jilt the gym and have a bedroom workout instead. Treat yourself and your partner to candlelit dinner, slow dancing, a romantic film – corny clichés, maybe, but they work. And, remember that sex can be fantastically soporific, making you more likely to get a good night's uninterrupted shut eye.

44. Stress 'n' relax

There's nothing wrong with stress: we're designed for it. The problem is how we deal with it.

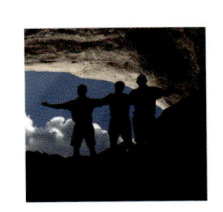

Coping with stress should be simple, the central message being simply: get stressed, then relax. So, why are we facing an epidemic of stress? The answer lies in the way we interpret the word 'relax'.

After beating off a tiger, or running away from it, our cavemen ancestors would have made their way back to the cave for a little lie down. There wasn't much to do in the caves so it was rest, calm and peace, and lots of sleep. Rest is essential to repair and recover from the effect of stress hormones on our organs.

But what do we do now after a stressful day? We might celebrate with alcohol, cigarettes, coffee (all of which trigger another stress response). Or, even worse, after a stressful situation, we jump straight into another one. This means that our bodies are bathed in stress hormones for far longer than was ever intended.

The body's hormones work in delicate balance. When the three

Defining idea...

'In times of stress be bold and valiant.'
HORACE

Here's an idea for you...

Next time you're waiting in a queue, or for traffic lights to change, see it as an opportunity for a mini-break. Do some deep breathing exercises and feel the tension flow out of your body.

main stress hormones – adrenaline, noradrenaline and cortisol – are fired, they affect the levels of all the others, notably insulin (which regulates sugar levels and energy) and serotonin (which affects mood and sleep). When they go awry over long periods of time, the results can be disastrous for our mental and physical health. This is why we start off stressed and end up stressed, fat, unhappy and unhealthy. The solution is to build relaxation in to your life, hour by hour, day by day.

See your day not as a long purgatory of stress but as lots of small stress responses punctuated with mini-relaxation breaks. For example, each waking hour should have five minutes of pleasure. So, after every hour of working, take a break to do something pleasurable – stretch, have a cuppa, daydream. Practise active relaxation for fifteen minutes every day – listening to music, yoga, sex, dancing. TV is passive and doesn't count. Spend three hours every week doing something you love. It should be calming, and non-work orientated. Only you can judge whether it is truly relaxing, so be honest with yourself in your choice.

45. There for you

Isolation worsens depression, but good friends can raise low moods. Discover the restorative powers of relationships.

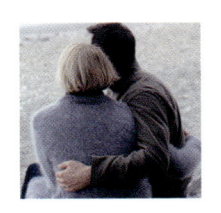

Are hugs the new drugs? Could a natter over coffee with a friend help your depression as much as pills or therapy? In the 1970s, sociologist George Brown paired up with psychiatrist Tirrel Harris and interviewed over a thousand women in Camberwell (a poor part of London). They found women with good, caring, intimate friendships were far less likely to get depressed. There's no reason to think this doesn't apply to guys too. The bottom line? Friendships are the single most effective safeguard against depression.

Harris carried on her ground-breaking work. Twenty years later, she studied another group of depressed women. They were randomly assigned to two groups. One group met a befriender; the other group was on a waiting list for one. Befrienders were volunteers acting as compassionate sounding-boards. They often met for chats over coffee. Nearly three-quarters of women with befrienders recovered from depression, compared with only 45% of those on the waiting list.

Defining idea...

'Friends are God's apology for relatives.'

HUGH KINGSMILL, British poet

Here's an idea for you...

Is your depression making you think you don't deserve friends? When you're down, being in company is almost always better than being alone, so, although you might not feel like going out, try to stay in touch with friends. If the phone seems too daunting, why not email, text or send postcards?

Remarkably, that's about the same success rate as drugs or therapy.

Even when you feel like staying home alone, remind yourself that seeing more of your friends lifts your mood. Just knowing someone cares about you can help. Confiding in close pals helps you think through why you're down. Good friends are usually great listeners and able to suggest viewpoints you hadn't thought of.

Some friends mean well but say useless things like, 'All you need is a new boyfriend'. Comments like this aren't usually malicious, so try just to filter them out. Take control by letting your friends know that telling you to 'snap out of it' or 'pull yourself together' actually makes things worse. Friends don't often know how to help, so you might need to spell it out by saying things like 'When you go out, it would be helpful if you'd invite me'.

46. Time to play

Picture what you'd do if you had a whole hour each day to yourself to spend doing exactly what you wanted.

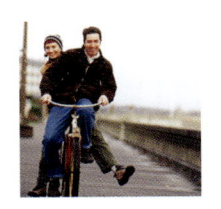

The 'desirable' things we'd like to spend an hour doing fall into two categories: the stuff we yearn to do because it's relaxing and fun and the stuff that's usually prefixed with a sense of 'ought to' because we know the rewards are worth it.

In the first category is lying in bed watching a movie; in the second, going for a run or quality time with the kids. We need to find the time for both, but both categories tend to get shunted into the sidings of our lives when life gets stressful. Exercise is one of the first things to go. How many times have you said 'I'd love to go to the gym – but I don't have the time'? So, ask yourself a big question: 'How will I feel in five years' time if I don't go?' More to the point – how will you look?

The same goes for 'life dreams', like writing a novel or learning Russian, which fall into the first category and add meaning to our lives. Nothing in your life will change unless you take

Defining idea...

'Life is what happens when we're busy doing something else.'
JOHN LENNON

Here's an idea for you...

Be creative in finding time for yourself. Take inspiration from a high-flying PR director who leaves for work to catch the 7.45 to work every morning. Except she doesn't have to catch the 7.45 – she catches the 8.15. She spends 30 minutes on the platform reading a novel. That's her break in the day.

action. People who spend at least some time doing the stuff that they want to do tend to feel that they're in control, and that's majorly destressing. So, how can we liberate our daily hour?

First get the big picture. Write down everything you're expected to make happen in the next month. Include everything. Look carefully: which items could you delegate to someone else? Be honest. Bet you that 10% can be offloaded. Now think about dumping 10% of what you have to do every day. Grade tomorrow's things-to-do list: A, must do; B, should do; C, could do. Now knock off a couple of Bs and three Cs. Add an activity that you know would destress you or add depth to your life and mark it with a whopping 'A'. Soon, you'll be prioritising yourself for at least an hour a day. Life really is too short to feel busy but achieve nothing that matters.

47. Imagine

Visualisation means using your mind to create pictures. Use it to relax or prepare yourself for action.

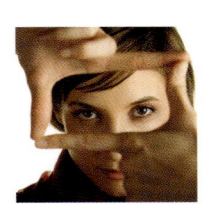

Creating pictures or scenes in your mind's eye is a great way to relax, but can be used in other ways as well. Have you ever thought 'What's the point? I'll only mess it up'? Instead of predicting how things are going to end up, why not visualise them the way you'd like them? Some people visualise their antidepressants as a waterfall, washing away depression. Or you can lift your mood by imagining yourself doing something you enjoy.

If you want to have a go, the best way to start is using visualisation techniques to relax. Find a quiet place where you won't be disturbed and close your eyes. Cast your mind back to a time in your life when you felt deeply relaxed. Imagine yourself in that calm place now. Try to bring it to life vividly, using all your senses. What can you see? Hear? Taste? Smell? Feel? Stay in that place as long as it takes to feel calm. It needs practice, but once you can picture your calming place, you've got an individualised, portable stress-buster. Creating pictures in your mind's eye

Defining idea...

'It is never too late to be what you might have been.'
GEORGE ELIOT

Here's an idea for you...

List possible solutions to your problems and imagine each solution is written on a door. Visualise yourself going through each door in turn. What do you find on the other side? If it's not what you'd like, cross back over the threshold and go through a different door.

can help you achieve things you never thought possible. Many people convince themselves that they'll fail exams. And guess what – they do. There's no surer route to failure than predicting it. Instead, spend five minutes a day during revision periods visualising the exam room. Imagine opening the paper and being pleased to see you could answer each question easily. Look forward to a positive outcome. Top athletes use visualisation during the last stages of training.

Similarly, visualisation can help you make a great first impression and maximise your impact in interviews. Dwelling on fears about rejection can make you overcautious and look defeated before you've even started. Instead, visualise wowing the panel with your answers, excelling at presentations, speaking fluently and articulately, and then being offered the job. Of course, no one can promise it will go like that on the day, but mental dress rehearsals will help you give your best performance.

Idea 48 – **You're worth it**

48. You're worth it

Down in the dumps with nothing to look forward too? Change that with some self-indulgent pampering.

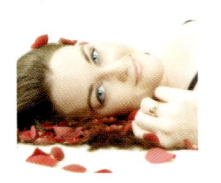

If your get up and go has got up and gone, this idea will give you the strength to go after it. When you're feeling the worse for wear some pampering and preening can be incredibly revitalising, raising your mood, confidence and self-esteem. When you wake up early and can't get back to sleep, don't lie there worrying, inject a little extra effort into your morning routine and reap daylong benefits.

Looking chic and sophisticated compared to dull and dreary makes a whopping difference to how people treat you and how you feel. Not convinced? How would you feel in response to these two statements? 'You look really tired. Are you OK?' 'Wow, you look amazing. Love the new suit.'

If you're strapped for cash right now, then perhaps it's time to check out some charity shops. You should be able to inject some pizzazz into your wardrobe on the cheap (and a fashion mistake that hasn't crippled

Defining idea...

'Happiness begins when one decides not to be something, but to be someone.'
COCO CHANEL

115

Here's an idea for you...

Perk yourself up with a pedicure. Relaxing foot massages can nurture, cleanse, energise and relax your body and mind.

your credit card is much easier to live with!). If the second-hand pickings are slim were you live, then give eBay a whirl: there's lots of interesting clothing to be had out there in cyberspace.

Putting on make-up might be the last thing you feel like doing when you're depressed, but the old saying 'outer beauty, inner strength' has a lot of truth in it. Researchers investigated the effects of make-up on our moods by giving daily makeovers to elderly people suffering from incontinence. Three months into the experiment, a third of them were out of their incontinence pads. Make-up helped them recover their dignity and sense of worth. Many hospitals employ beauticians to improve the well-being of cancer patients.

When you're fed up or feeling fusty, half an hour at your hairdresser is great for hauling up your humour. Many hairdressers have first-rate listening skills. A humble cut and blow dry can turn into an impromptu therapy session. The lift you get might not last longer than your retouched roots, but it could become a highlight of your month.

49. Shades of grey

Depressed people think in all-or-nothing terms. Don't let self-imposed perfectionism make you feel you never measure up.

Most things aren't major disasters or cause for great celebration. Life tends to throw us a mixture of pain and pleasure. When you're depressed, you can easily lose perspective on this as depression often makes us think in all-or-nothing terms. One depressed patient ran the London marathon. Because he didn't come first in his running club, he felt there had been no point taking part. Does self-imposed perfectionism mean you never measure up?

Experts call this black-and-white thinking. And far from just being a sign of depression, it worsens it, dragging you lower and lower. Black-and-white thinking makes you feel more depressed, worried, stressed or angry. It also stops you from doing things that'd help you feel better, like seeing friends.

Seeing the world without shades of grey is a primitive form of self-protection. For example, if there's a fire, you're more likely to survive if

Defining idea...

'Life is not a spelling bee where one mistake wipes out all the things we have done right.'
RABBI HAROLD S. KUSHNER

Here's an idea for you...

Start keeping track of times you use the words 'always', 'never', 'completely' or 'typical'. Get into the habit of asking yourself if you could be exaggerating. Perhaps you're only focusing on things that have gone wrong and forgetting all the stuff you've achieved. Do you become so absorbed in your weaknesses that you forget your strengths? Are you assuming you can't do anything to change things? It's time to stop losing sleep over the way things used to be: focus on how they are now.

you make a snap decision to get out than if you hang around weighing up pros and cons of various exit routes. So it's great for life-threatening crises, but not so hip or hot for everyday stuff. The more your thoughts are polarised into extremes, the more your moods will swing like a pendulum.

'Nothing helps.' 'I'll never feel better.' 'It'll be terrible.' 'What's the point trying?' 'I've got to get it completely right.' If any of these phrases sound familiar, you've become a victim of the black-and-white thoughts squad. Recognising this has happened is a major step. However, like anything new, moving from all-or-nothing to shades of grey can be hard. You need to believe in options, compromise or middle ground.

Think back to the last time you used black-and-white thinking. What thoughts went through your mind? How did you feel afterwards? You can't always control how you feel, but you can control these all-or-nothing thoughts.

50. Memory fix

Never lose your keys again. Here's why stress eats your memory – and what you can do about it.

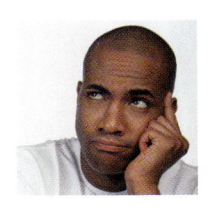

Often you can't remember where you left the car keys. Sometimes you can't remember where you left the car. Memory lapses aren't necessarily the first indication of Alzheimer's, so don't worry. But if they are increasing in frequency, it could be that your memory is a casualty of a hectic lifestyle. This adds to your stress.

The only answer is to be aware that when you're busy and stressed you're not taking in information in the same way and you're not going to be able to recall it. Make like a boy scout and be prepared. For example, on a busy day when you meet someone new, be aware that you are more likely to forget their name. Make more effort than usual during introductions. Repeat a new name inside your head. Use it again in conversation as soon as you can.

When learning anything new during a stressed period, repeat it to yourself and if possible say it out loud three or four times, increasing the amount of time between each repetition. The

Defining idea...

'Happiness is nothing more than good health and a bad memory.'
ALBERT SCHWEITZER

Here's an idea for you...

Try supplements. There's some evidence that the herb gingko biloba improves blood flow to the brain and hence memory. You can buy supplements containing gingko at chemists and health food shops. Sage is also good for memory.

'repetition-pause-repetition' pattern strengthens memory. This technique also works for items or tasks that you have to remember – and always forget. If you're fed up going to the supermarket to buy tomatoes and coming back with everything else but tomatoes, try it. If it doesn't work, then make allowances and leave notes in your purse or on your toothbrush – places where you will certainly check. Don't rely on your memory.

What few people realise is that most routine actions will cause memory problems if you do them differently every day. That's because, for instance, when you put items you use frequently in different places from one day to the next, you have to block the memory of what you did with them yesterday, and the day before, in order to find them today. This is why you've spent hours looking for your keys or wallet. The answer is to create a memory pot – a bowl or basket near your front door where everything goes as soon as you get home, and which you check before you leave the house.

51. A bright future

Sadly, once depression has paid you a visit, it's likely to return. Recognise its calling card and send it packing.

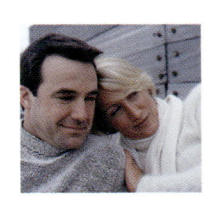

Many people wonder how they'll manage after stopping drugs or therapy. Well, here's how. Think back to when you last became depressed and analyse specifically what was going on at the time, how you were feeling and, with hindsight, the first things you noticed that were different. The signs vary widely. Elliot, who usually struggles to get up, starts waking up early. Janine, a real foodie, loses interest in cooking and her appetite dwindles.

If you're finding it difficult to recognise any warning signs yourself, why not recruit some help? People you live with are often good at noticing subtle signs and friends can be a good bet too. Once you identify depression's forewarning, you'll be able to stop it in its tracks.

Think ahead over the next year and identify any events that are likely to trigger depression. Maybe your daughter is leaving home or your dad is getting very frail. It doesn't have to

Defining idea...

'I like living. I have sometimes been wildly, despairingly, acutely miserable, racked with sorrow, but through it all I still know that just to be alive is a grand thing.'
AGATHA CHRISTIE

Here's an idea for you...

Make sure you see supportive friends and family: they can be a key to defeating depression. Divvy up responsibilities and let them help you with overwhelming tasks. Inevitably, you'll think back to last time you were depressed, but instead of dwelling on how terrible things were, try to consider what helped you feel better last time. If you can keep some sort of routine going, so much the better.

be anything major, though, and for many people it might be post-holiday blues. Although you can't avoid events that could set off depression, at least you can plan around them.

Once you've identified warning signs and potentially tricky times, come up with a battle plan. To do this, it really is vital to reflect on what you learnt before that has worked for you. Interrogate yourself about what you can do to build on what you've learned: What helped you get better? What ideas will you use next time? What would lessen its impact? Who else can help you? It's a good idea to jot your best answers down. They're a kind of first-aid kit to keep the initial flush of sadness away.

52. On the shelf

Find out what's in the pharm yard. Which drugs work; which make you feel worse; how can you tell the difference?

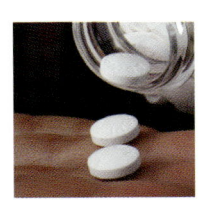

Not sure if antidepressants are for you? They're best at busting so-called biological symptoms: changes in sleep pattern, lost appetite, feeling slowed down or agitated, concentration problems and feeling like your sex drive has driven off somewhere. It takes up to four weeks for antidepressants to start working. Yep, faster than therapy, but tablets won't teach you how to stop thinking depressing thoughts, help you understand why you feel bad, or find a better rate mortgage. Here's a breakdown of the key players you might encounter. Let's think of them as tribes, where members work in similar ways and have comparable side effects. Because each tribe member is slightly different, it means if one doesn't help, another from the same tribe might.

Tribe: Tricyclic antidepressants (TCAs).
Members: Amitriptyline, clomipramine, dothiepine, imipramine, trimipramine, lofepramine.
Myth: Old, obsolete and ought to be left on the shelf.
Reality: An old tribe but they're as effective as any newbie.
Best bits: Can make you feel sleepy so they're great for insomniacs.

Worst bits: Lots of side effects so the dose has to be upped slowly. Can give you a dry mouth, constipation, blurred vision and drowsiness, so no school run. Very dangerous in overdose so professionals don't give them to suicidal people.

Tribe: Selective serotonin reuptake inhibitors (SSRIs).
Members: Fluoxetine (Prozac), fluvoxamine, paroxetine, sertraline, citalopram.
Myth: Mind-altering, euphoria-inducing party pills that ought to be added to our water supply.
Reality: Choosy about which chemical receptors they'll hook up with so there are few side effects.
Best bits: Won't leave you with a dry mouth or fuzzy head.
Worst bits: Nausea is pretty common in the first few weeks. Can wreak havoc with your love life by delaying your ability to orgasm. Might sound like fun, but gets exasperating.

Tribe: Selective noradrenaline reuptake inhibitors (SNRIs).
Member: Reboxetine.
Myth: Newbie sponsored by footwear manufacturers.
Reality: Acts on brain chemical noradrenaline, vital for that perky, zest-for-life feeling.
Best bits: Helps you get going if your motivation's low.
Worst bits: Some people get dry mouths, constipation, drowsiness and feel light-headed.

Brilliant ideas

Tribe: Monoamine oxidase inhibitors (MAOIs).
Members: Phenelzine, selegiline, isocarboxacid.
Myth: Stuffy old tribe with too many rules.
Reality: Oldest antidepressants that were left on the shelf but are now making a comeback because they often work where other tribes have failed.
Best bits: Good for what the trade calls atypical depression, a fancy name for comfort eating, oversleeping, being irritable and feeling hypersensitive.
Worst bits: Masses of food restrictions. You could suffer a blood pressure hike which can cause a stroke if you eat anything from a long list that includes cheese, anything with yeast (including beer), red wine and pickled herrings. The same reaction happens with many over-the-counter drugs.

Tribe: Reversible inhibitors of monoamine oxidase type A (RIMAs).
Members: Moclobemide.
Myth: Old pills in new packets.
Reality: A better, safer MAOI.
Best bits: Few side effects and no food restrictions.
Worst bits: Insomnia, dizziness and headaches.

Here's an idea for you...

Confusingly, all drugs have more than one name. To investigate more about them, check out the universal generic name – for instance, phenelzine. Manufacturers give a trade name, like Nardil, which is often different in different countries. This is annoying for everyone except the marketing bozos because it's easier to sell a drug called damnitall than pleboxyflymoxyethymethylamine. The best-known trade name is Prozac – once the new kid on the antidepressant block, now one of its stars.

Tribe: Noradrenaline and selective serotonin reuptake inhibitors (NASSAs).
Members: Mirtazepine.
Myth: Antidepressants for astronauts.
Reality: Often refreshes the parts other tribes haven't reached.
Best bits: May have an effect more quickly than other tribes.
Worst bits: Avoid alcohol, as it may make you more sleepy.
Tribe: Dual uptake inhibitor.
Members: Venlafaxine, milnacipran.
Myth: TCAs rebadged.
Reality: The best of TCAs without their hassles.
Best bits: Works quickly.
Worst bits: Nightmares, loss of interest in sex.

Defining idea...

'The idea of throwing away my depression, of having to create a whole way of living and being, of having to create a whole new personality that did not contain misery as its leitmotif was daunting. Now, with the help of a biochemical cure, it was going to go away.'

ELIZABETH WURTZEL, *Prozac Nation*

Brilliant ideas

This book is published by Infinite Ideas, creators of the acclaimed **52 Brilliant Ideas series**. If you found this book helpful, there are other titles in the **Brilliant Little Ideas** series which you may also find of interest.

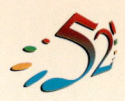

- **Be incredibly creative:** 52 brilliant little ideas to hone your mind
- **Catwalk looks:** 52 brilliant little ideas to look gorgeous always
- **Drop a dress size:** 52 brilliant little ideas to lose weight and stay slim
- **Find your dream job:** 52 brilliant little ideas for total career happiness
- **Heal your troubled mind:** 52 brilliant little ideas for tackling stress and defeating depression
- **Healthy children's lunches:** 52 brilliant little ideas for junk-free meals kids will love
- **Incredible sex:** 52 brilliant little ideas to take you all the way
- **Make your money work:** 52 brilliant little ideas for rescuing your finances
- **Perfect romance:** 52 brilliant little ideas for finding and keeping a lover
- **Raising young children:** 52 brilliant little ideas for parenting under 5s
- **Relax:** 52 brilliant little ideas to chill out
- **Shape up your bum:** 52 brilliant little ideas for maximising your gluteus

For more detailed information on these books and others published by Infinite Ideas please visit www.infideas.com.

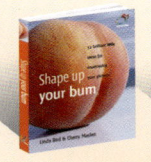

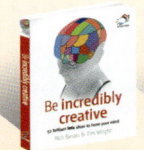

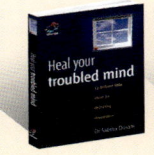

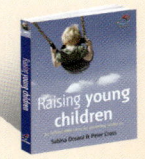

See reverse for order form.

52 Brilliant Ideas – **Heal your troubled mind**

Qty	Title	RRP
	Be incredibly creative	£5.99
	Catwalk looks	£5.99
	Drop a dress size	£5.99
	Find your dream job	£5.99
	Heal your troubled mind	£5.99
	Healthy children's lunches	£5.99
	Incredible sex	£5.99
	Make your money work	£5.99
	Perfect romance	£5.99
	Raising young children	£5.99
	Relax	£5.99
	Shape up your bum	£5.99
	Add £2.49 postage per delivery address	
	Final TOTAL	

Name: ....

Delivery address: ....

....

....

E-mail:...............................Tel (in case of problems): ....

By post Fill in all relevant details, cut out or copy this page and send along with a cheque made payable to Infinite Ideas. Send to: *Brilliant Little Ideas*, Infinite Ideas, 36 St Giles, Oxford OX1 3LD. **Credit card orders over the telephone** Call +44 (0) 1865 514 888. Lines are open 9am to 5pm Monday to Friday.

Please note that no payment will be processed until your order has been dispatched. Goods are dispatched through Royal Mail within 14 working days, when in stock. We never forward personal details on to third parties or bombard you with junk mail. The prices quoted are for UK and RoI residents only. If you are outside these areas please contact us for postage and packing rates. Any questions or comments please contact us on 01865 514 888 or email info@infideas.com.